Elemental Medicine

Learn it for Life!

Copyright ©2013 by John Bielinski, Jr., MS, PA

This edition published by CME4Life and "Who's Your PAPPA" Productions, East Amherst, New York. Printed by Parrinello Printing Inc., Cheektowaga, New York

The author, editor and publisher have made every effort to provide accurate information. However, they are not responsible for errors, omissions, or for any outcomes related to the use and content of this book and take no responsibility for the use of the products and procedures described. Treatments and side effects described in this book may not be applicable to all people; likewise, some people may require a dose or experience a side effect that is not described herein. Drugs and medical devices are discussed that may have limited availability controlled by the Food and Drug Administration (FDA) for use only in a research study or clinical trial. Research, clinical practice and government regulations often change the accepted standard in this field. When consideration is being given to use of any drug in the clinical setting, the health care provider or reader is responsible for determining FDA status of the drug, reading the package insert and reviewing prescribing information for the most up-to-date recommendations on dose, precautions, and contraindications, and determining the appropriate usage for the product. This is especially important in the case of drugs that are now or seldom used.

Editor: Loriann Kostusiak
Design & Layout: Deb Wilby
Cover Photograph: Cassie Brown

First Edition

ISBN 978-0-9892209-0-3

Library of Congress Cataloging-in-Publication Data
Bielinski, John Jr., MS, PA
Elemental Medicine-Learn it for Life - 1st Edition
Manufactured in the United States of America

Elemental Medicine

Learn it for Life

John Bielinski Jr., MS, PA

To my wife and family
Michelle, Johnny, Matthew and Sarah

God's speed, Plant seeds

TABLE OF CONTENTS

My intention with this book was never to make it a referenced-based, scientific approach to evidence-based medicine. We learn and study evidence-based medicine, but as practitioners, we also need the art of medicine. You can approach a patient from a purely textbook perspective. If you practice the art of medicine, however, you recognize the subtleties of disease presentation, listen carefully to factors in patient's lives, and know your limits of knowledge so that you can ask for help when you need it.

As medical providers, we must be constantly open to learning. We must challenge and expand our medical knowledge, deepen our understanding and perception of human beings, and constantly reevaluate and fine-tune our effectiveness as caretakers.

My hope is that this book serves as a catalyst to your growth. My goal is to share my knowledge and experience so that you may be inspired to see an alternate perspective and seek a deeper understanding of the way you practice medicine. As a community of medical providers, we care for each other's families: wives, husbands, children, sisters, brothers, parents and friends. Every single time we approach a patient, we must do so with this in mind, and care, as we would want another medical professional to care for our loved ones.

Thank you for reading.

John Bielinski

CHAPTER 1

THE COMPLETE BLOOD COUNT

The CBC is the most basic of the labs that we order. It is a primary screener of disease and a basic monitoring of the patient. The CBC gives an idea of the body's response to stress, the body's oxygen carrying capacities as well as giving a platelet count, which reveals how well the blood is clotting. There are two main elements that we need to evaluate when looking at a CBC. We are going to look at the formed elements, which are red blood cells, white blood cells and platelets, and we are also going to look at the indices, which are used to describe the red blood cell count and then give us a gauge of disease.

When we talk about the formed elements, let's start off talking about the white blood cell, also known as a leukocyte, where an abnormal elevation of white blood cells is referred to as a leukocytosis, and an abnormally low white blood cell count is referred to as leukopenia. There are two reasons why we would have a leukocytosis, and it is really best to find whether there is an infectious problem or a noninfectious problem. There are three ways to gage infection from a CBC. We are concerned with the absolute number of white blood cells, the percentage of neutrophils and the number of immature cells. The absolute number of white blood cells means the total number of white blood cells. A normal value is between 5,000 and 10,000. When we look at someone for an infection, the first thing we are going to look at is the absolute number. Is this a white count of 12,000, or 14,000, or 24,000? That will give us a clue as to whether the cause of the problem is, indeed, infection.

When it comes to white blood cells, there are five different kinds. We have neutrophils, basophils, lymphocytes, monocytes, and eosinophils. Neutrophils encompass approximately 75% of all the white blood cells put together. So, neutrophils are the powerhouses that are in charge of the phagocytosis of bacteria. When we have a bacterial infection, neutrophils have a tendency to increase in number. So, when we denote a patient whom we feel has an infection, we would denote their absolute number of white blood cells, let's say 17,000. Also, we would note the number of neutrophils. If a patient has a 17,000 white count and 90% neutrophils, it strongly suggests a bacterial infection. So, neutrophils are really the white blood cell count we are most interested in. Next, when I talk about immature cells being noted, I am talking about band cells. Band cells are immature white blood cells, and I like to suggest that they are similar to the United States Marines, which means if you see a bunch of United States Marines in a county, you know there has been a bad fight that has gone on, and normally the Marines are the first to go in, the first to fight. Band cells suggest that a pretty intense infection has been going on and has used up all the white blood cells (the neutrophils) that are available to the body and the body has had to call on immature cells to come in and help fight the battle. In summary, there are three ways to gauge infection from a CBC: the white blood cell count, the neutrophil count, and the band count.

Now, how do we work up infection? We have a patient who comes that we believe may have some degree of infection, and classically this could be a nursing home patient who is demented and really cannot give us much of a history, or even a child who is sick, and may have an infection. So, how do we work up infection, and how do we use the white blood cell count to help us determine whether this is a patient has an infectious problem or noninfectious problem? The first step is to use all resources available to get a good history, whether it is from nursing home staff or a parent.

In addition to a thorough history, we need objective findings, including vital signs. We need to get a valid temperature, and the best way to do that is to get a rectal temperature. Axillary temperature and tympanic temperature are often inaccurate. Oral temperature could be valid if you have a compliant patient who can hold the thermometer under the tongue with mouth closed. But still, there is variability in how that temperature is obtained. If you want the best, valid temperature, get a rectal temperature. Now, do I do that in all my patients? No, of course I don't. If a 30-year-old female comes in with probable pneumonia, I don't do a rectal temperature. But, as a medical provider you are solely responsible for your patient's health, and the most valid way to know if they have a fever or not is with a rectal temperature. The second thing we have to consider is that 9 out of 10 infectious problems that would hit the average adult, or child, would be an infection in the wind or the water, wind being pneumonia and water being urine. You need to do a two-view chest x-ray and a urinalysis with culture. Now, a two-view chest x-ray is important because we can see lower into the lungs and behind the heart, which may be missed on a one-view chest x-ray. So, always do a two-view chest x-ray and a urine.

The second aspect of objective findings are basic screening labs. This would include first the white blood cell count where we would look at the absolute number, the number of neutrophils and the number of bands. Second would be blood cultures x2. Let's focus on cultures. Staphylococcus is a very common germ that resides on our skin, in our nares, in our axilla and in our groin. When we do cultures on a person, we draw them from the arm, and if the blood cultures grow out staph, we would have to be concerned about whether this is a bacterial infection that is in the blood. So, is this patient bacteremic with staph or was it just a contamination from the skin? A way to avoid confusion is to get two sets of blood cultures by either drawing from two separate sites (having the nurse draw from the right arm and from the left arm) or drawing from the same site but half an hour apart. Blood cultures should be a provider's knee-jerk response to working up infection. At times they may have a low clinical yield, but just do blood cultures. From my experience, I have found myself in hot water at times working up infection where I did not first do blood cultures. Now, this does have to do with hospital administration and with reimbursement costs. If you are working up someone for infection, especially pneumonia, do one set of blood cultures. It is important to get two sets of cultures when you think you have a patient who is truly septic, looks sick, has a high fever, borderline blood pressure and is shaking with rigors. If you really think the patient is sick, order blood cultures. Now, under those circumstances, you would not want to wait a half hour between blood draws because you would want to draw blood and get cultures quickly so you can get antibiotics on board. In that case, I would recommend using two different sites.

If 9 out of 10 infections are from wind or water, we have to be concerned with the abdomen and the cerebral spinal fluid as that 1 out of 10 cause for infection. Let's talk about the abdomen. Physical exam of the abdomen has to do with guarding, rebound and rigidity. In looking at the pathophysiology of the abdomen, there are the intestines, held in place by the peritoneum. When the peritoneum becomes irritated, it clamps down and clamps the muscle structures down. The only way to really get good at determining whether a patient has peritonitis (inflammation of the peritoneum) is by feeling a lot of bellies and feeling surgical bellies (a patient who has peritonitis).

Guarding is the response that occurs when, as you examine a patient's belly, they voluntarily flex their stomach muscles so you cannot examine them. If you want a good example of this, especially if you are a girl, go up to a guy in a bar and grab his biceps. Now, what a guy will typically do is he will flex his biceps voluntarily, kind of saying, "Hey, my arm is always strong, I'm a strong guy." That is guarding, and you document that as positive localized guarding in the right lower quadrant. Rigidity is an unresponsive flexing of stomach muscles, where you cannot get him to relax or distract him so you can examine the belly because the muscles are constantly flexed. That is known as a rigid abdomen. Rebound tenderness has to do with actually shaking the peritoneum, and that shaking causes pain. Now, from the physical exam perspective, as I am sure you folks know, you push down on one part of the belly, you let go, and that let go vibrates the peritoneum which causes pain at the site of irritation. Another way to do this is to do a heel jar test. This is where I would approach a patient from the bedside, make a closed fist and actually strike the heel of the foot a number of times. This will shake the peritoneum and cause pain at the site of inflammation. From an historical perspective, this is where you would ask the patient, "Did every bump on the car ride over cause you pain?" Now, every bump that is hit would vibrate the belly, again, causing a degree of rebound tenderness.

With regard to the abdominal exam, rebound, guarding and rigidity, when you are dealing with a patient who has diabetes or who is on chronic steroids, all bets on the physical exam are off. In a patient with diabetes, the nerves that integrate the peritoneum are kind of blunted, so they will not have normal physical exam findings. It is the same thing in a patient on chronic steroids.

When it comes to the cerebral spinal fluid, we should be very concerned about meningitis. Any patient that you evaluate for an infection, for the rest of your career, must be given a neck evaluation. A person coming in with a fever is very different than a person who comes in with a fever and a rigid neck. Now, the neck exam of someone who has meningitis is not like someone who slept in a funny position and woke up having a sore neck. A rigid neck is when someone's neck is board-like. They cannot turn their head to look over their shoulder without causing tremendous pain. Their body twists at the shoulders to compensate for that pain. Physical exam findings include Brudzinski sign, where you actually flex the neck bringing the chin down to the chest, which causes severe pain down the back. Kernig sign is when the patient is on their back, supine, and you have them flex at the knee and at the hip. When you extend at the knee, it causes severe pain in the lower back because it is pulling on the meninges. These are also known as meningeal signs.

The red blood cells have a lifespan of approximately 120 days. When we talk about red blood cells, we are concerned with three related values: the absolute number of red blood cells, the hemoglobin, and the hematocrit. Now, the absolute value of red blood cells is used to calculate hemoglobin and hematocrit, and it is the hemoglobin and hematocrit that we use to make clinical decisions. Out of the three numbers that we use to help us gage a patient's oxygen carrying capacity, we are really concerned with the hemoglobin and hematocrit, which are derived from the red blood cell count. Now, the hemoglobin is the oxygen-carrying component of a red blood cell, and it is measured in grams per deciliter. Normal is approximately 13 through 15. When the hematocrit is a measured percentage of a spun-down sample, a normal percentage is about 42 to 52%. Now, when it comes to hemoglobin to hematocrit, there is a very fixed ratio of 1:3, where if the hemoglobin is 10, the hematocrit is 30. Or, if the hemoglobin is 13, then the hematocrit is 39. Of interest is that some medical schools train people to really focus on one value when other medical schools train people to focus on the other. Like, I am a hematocrit guy, and I think of patients in terms of hematocrit. If someone called me on the phone and said, "Hey, I'm sending in a patient who has a hemoglobin of 7," I have a tough time relating that hemoglobin of 7 to clinical use. I have to convert this over to 21, and I have a good idea of how a patient will look with a hematocrit of 21. Other people will use hemoglobin, and if I say, "Hey, I have a patient with a hematocrit of 30," they are going to translate over to hemoglobin. So, with that said, when you are in a hospital or when you are working with a physician, use both. Give them the hemoglobin and hematocrit even though they both kind of are relative to each other, but different people think in terms of different numbers.

When we look at red blood cells, we are really looking to see whether this patient has anemia. That is the primary reason why we look at the hemoglobin and hematocrit. Now, anemia is not a disease. It is a symptom of a disease. A little boy can have a fever, and that does not really tell you anything about how sick he is. It could just be a virus or could be bacterial pneumonia. It is the same thing with a patient who is anemic. Anemia is a sign of a disease, and we need to figure out why they have anemia. It shows a degree of not thinking through the disease properly if you just say, "Hey, I have a patient who is anemic," without saying why. Whether it is iron-deficiency anemia or a gastrointestinal bleed that is the cause. So, you should never in your career say just, "I have a patient who is anemic." It is more helpful to say, "I have a patient with anemia of unknown etiology," because you have not quite figured it out yet.

How will a patient with anemia look? As I have said earlier, a normal hematocrit value is between 42 and 50. So, if I ask the question, "How will a patient look with a hematocrit of 25, and what clinical findings would a patient have with a hematocrit of 25? The answer is, "It depends." The symptoms of anemia are based on the onset or the rapidity, how rapid the onset was of the anemia. If you have someone who has sickle cell anemia and their anemia has developed over years, the body will have compensated very well for a hematocrit of 25, and these people could be a bit fatigued at times, but overall they go through their daily functions without any limitations. If somebody has been in a car accident and has lacerated their spleen, and they go from a hematocrit of 45 to 25 in a matter of an hour, they would be knocking on death's door. So, when you say someone is anemic at 25, the symptoms of the anemia are based on the onset.

A question I am often asked by students is, "At what number do we do a blood transfusion on a patient?" Is it 25, is 20? When do we transfuse? My answer to this question is really not concrete. A rough gage is to say a hematocrit of 25, but that is really relative to how long it took the patient to get there and what signs and symptoms are present from anemia. So, this question we will answer more in the chapter when we talk specifically about blood transfusions. Understand that anemia and transfusion is more of an art than a science, and it is very practitioner-dependent. A surgeon may be very quick to transfuse at a hematocrit of 25, but an internist may be a whole lot more sluggish to do that, or even visa versa.

When we evaluate anemia, the most important thing we need to look at to determine what is causing the anemia is the size of the cell or the mean corpuscular volume (MCV). You can have small cells, you can have normal cells or you can have large cells, all dependent on the MCV. Normal MCV is between 81 and 97, so if you have an MCV of 70, you have small cells. An MCV of 105 indicates large cells. Let's focus on microcytic anemia. Now, there are four main causes of microcytic anemia, and I hope these STIC with you.

S	**SIDEROBLASTIC**
T	**THALASSEMIA**
I	**IRON-DEFICIENCY**
C	**CHRONIC DISEASE**

The S stands for sideroblastic. This has to do with heavy

metal ingestion such as lead. (When we are evaluating the relatively uncommon sideroblastic anemia, know that a buzzword on your board exam is "basophilic stippling.") The T stands for thalassemia, which would be diagnosed by hemoglobin electrophoresis. This is most often seen in people of Mediterranean descent and can be anything from a minor trait and relatively insignificant to the patient, to a major trait meaning they do not live a long life. The I is for iron-deficiency. The C stands for chronic disease. Anemia of chronic disease is more of a diagnosis of exclusion, and this may also be normocytic. As a patient ages and has multiple medical problems, they are found to have a degree of anemia, and when they are worked up, there is really no cause found. Therefore, providers will say, "Well, it is just anemia of chronic disease and pretty close to their baseline."

The red blood cells are stimulated by erythropoietin. No erythropoietin is created from the kidneys. A patient who has renal insufficiency or renal failure and is on dialysis will have very low erythropoietin levels and will be anemic. It is quite common for someone on dialysis to have anemia, secondary to decreased erythropoietin. Patients who are severely anemic from this etiology will receive erythropoietin shots from time to time.

The most common reason why someone would have microcytic anemia is from gastrointestinal bleeding. This could be from an ulcer in the stomach or duodenum, a polyp or a malignancy in the lower gastrointestinal tract. Now, the cells that are produced in response to bleeding come out smaller than the red blood cells that are there physiologically. When we are concerned a patient has gastrointestinal bleeding, the first thing we have to do is a rectal exam. If this is positive for blood, then a lot of our work up is done and we can refer on to the gastroenterologist.

To clinch the diagnosis of gastrointestinal bleeding, there are a couple of tests that we can look at on the CBC that would be helpful. The first one is the MCV. Now, the mien corpuscular volume again has to do with the size of the cells. As I have stated before, the red blood cell's lifespan is 120 days. So, just for the purpose of understanding, let's say it is about 100 days. So, if you go with saying the red blood cell lives approximately 100 days, we could make the assumption that every day 1% of our red blood cells are turned over. Now if someone is having gastrointestinal bleeding, the cells that are produced in response to the bleeding come out smaller. The MCV is an average of all the red blood cells. If you have someone who has been bleeding for 10 days, it means 10% of their cells are going to be smaller, and the MCV will not have changed. It will still look normalized because 90% of the cells are of normal size. The MCV will not change to a microcytic state until approximately half the cells are small. So, if half the cells would have to be small to change the MCV, this bleeding (based on using 100 days as the lifespan) would take 50 days for the cells to become microcytic. Therefore, if you have someone who comes in with a microcytic anemia from gastrointestinal bleeding, it is safe to assume that this bleeding has been going on approximately two months or greater. If you have a young lady who comes in with vaginal bleeding that has been going on for two weeks, and you check the hemoglobin and hematocrit, which are 10 and 30, it is lower than her baseline. And, if the MCV is normal, it is consistent with someone who has had bleeding going on two weeks.

Another helpful test to determine if someone is having gastrointestinal bleeding is a reticulocyte count. A reticulocyte is an immature red blood cell, synonymous with the band's cell as the white blood cells count, as the reticulocyte is to a red blood cell. Reticulocytes come out only when red blood cells are disappearing. This is either through gastrointestinal bleeding or hemolysis. Normally when you check someone's blood, the reticulocyte count is approximately 1-2%. If someone is having gastrointestinal bleeding, or hemolysis, the reticulocyte count will be up to 4-5%. So, a helpful test to work up someone you presume is having gastrointestinal bleeding is a reticulocyte count. If this is high, they are having blood loss, and 49 out of 50 times, it is from gastrointestinal bleeding or some kind of bleeding. It is a relatively inexpensive test. It requires the lab technician to just stain the smear in a slightly different way. So, it is a helpful test and is relatively inexpensive.

Another part of the CBC that is helpful in working up a patient with anemia is the red blood cell distribution width (RDW). The RDW is a bit confusing. The bottom line is that it is helpful to determine early gastrointestinal bleeding. The red blood cell distribution width has to do with looking at the difference between the biggest cell and the smallest cell in giving you a percentage. Now, normally, someone who is not bleeding has a difference between their small cell and biggest cell at about 10%, so that is a normal variation; a normal red blood cell distribution width. As I said earlier, when someone is bleeding, the cells that come out in response to that bleeding will be disproportionally small. So, if you have a red blood cell distribution width that is 15 or 20%, it means the difference in the smallest cell to the biggest cell is higher than baseline and that suggests early gastrointestinal bleeding. So, if you have that girl who had vaginal bleeding for a week or two, and you check her H&H which is low, her MCV is normal, you can expect the RDW to be high. So, again, if we are using 1% turnover of red blood cells daily, after two weeks, you can assume that approximately 14% of her red blood cells would be small. Now, that is not enough to change the MCV to a microcytic status, but it is enough to enlarge the RDW. Now, here is a question for you? How will the reticulocyte count look in a girl who is having vaginal bleeding for the past two weeks? It would be elevated because of blood loss.

Now let's talk about macrocytic anemia. These are people who have large cells and who are anemic. In macrocytic anemia, the most common by far is B-12 or folate deficiency. If someone comes in with a macrocytic anemia, we have to check a B-12 and folate level. Also, this is a good time to pick up someone who is an alcoholic. These people can have what is called a "martini macrocytosis." They have large cells, but may not always be anemic. If someone comes in with macrocytosis, you should be concerned that they have a history of excessive drinking. The liver has about two years' store of B12, So, if someone comes in B12 deficient, it has taken a long time to get to that level. You basically check a B12 level. If someone comes in with folate deficiency, it can happen in about two months, or about the same time frame it takes to have a gastrointestinal bleed and become microcytic. So, folate can happen in about two months whereas B12 deficiency takes years.

In summary, a typical anemia work up is done in the following steps. If a patient is anemic, the first question we have to ask is, "How does the MCV look?" Do we have a patient who is microcytic, normocytic or macrocytic? If they are microcytic, order a reticulocyte count. If it is high, we know that they have blood loss, either hemolysis or gastrointestinal bleeding. We would order iron studies and would have to do a rectal exam. So, someone who is microcytic, do a reticulocyte count, iron studies and a rectal exam. A patient who comes in who is normocytic, you would need to do a reticulocyte count, do a rectal exam (this is where we would evaluate red blood cell distribution width to help us identify an early gastrointestinal bleed) and this would be a good time to check renal functions to see if this is someone with renal insufficiency and not secreting enough erythropoietin. With a patient who has a macrocytic anemia, we do a B12 and folate level, and we have to get a very good history about their drinking. Are they a daily drinker or are they a closet drinker. Just be aware that people who are heavy alcoholics will not come clean and admit the exact degree of what they drink, so do not hesitate to get the family involved in the questioning.

Finally, I would like to discuss the indices and describe the red blood cells. The MCV is the mien corpuscular volume, which is the size of the red blood cells. The MCV is the most important index when it comes to working up a patient with anemia. The next one is the mien corpuscular hemoglobin or MCH, which refers to the color of the cell and is of low clinical value. A patient who is microcytic almost always would be considered hypochromic (MCH means they have small cells that are a little more pale). So, mien corpuscular hemoglobin refers to color. You will hear people referred to as having a macrocytic hyperchromic anemia, which means they have big cells that are dark. Again, the fact that they are dark or light is really irrelevant. We want to know the MCV. Are they small or are they big? MCHC stands for mien corpuscular hemoglobin concentration. This has no clinical value and no decisions can really be made based on the MCHC. The RDW (red blood cell distribution width) can be used to help us diagnose early gastrointestinal bleeding. It is not an absolute test and does not make me hang my hat on a diagnosis, but it is a helpful test. So, once again if someone comes in with a normocytic anemia and a high RDW, it suggests that the patient may be bleeding before the MCV has changed, and we really need to do rectal studies.

CHAPTER 2

THE BASIC CHEMISTRIES

The basic metabolic panel, also known as BMP, are the basic chemistries we order in screening someone for disease or monitoring disease. The basic chemistries include cations (sodium and potassium) anions (chloride and bicarbonate) and renal functions (BUN, creatinine, and glucose).

We are going to start off talking about sodium. There are some general truisms that you need to be aware of when looking at sodium. First, under normal physiology, that is if the patient is not sick and has normal mechanisms, sodium goes where water goes. So, if someone is retaining sodium, they are going retain water. If they are peeing out sodium, they are going to pee out water. Another truism is that sodium is the main osmole in blood by far. So, when it comes to the osmolality of our blood, sodium is the biggest player.

Someone who is hypernatremic is easy, *if it is high, they are dry*. It is just that simple. So, if someone is hypernatremic, they need intravenous fluids or oral fluids in general. *If it is high, they are dry*. Hyponatremia is a much more complicated work up, but, with a couple simple steps, it can help you feel much more confident in your diagnosis. The first step in the work up of hyponatremia is to check serum osmolality. As I said before, sodium is the number one osmole in the blood. So, if your number one osmole is very low, you would expect serum osmolality to be low as well. If serum osmolality is high, and the patient has low sodium, you have to make the assumption that there is some funky osmole in the blood that is throwing things off. By far, the most common is glucose. So, if you have a patient who comes in with a glucose level of 600 and a sodium of 124, we should expect that because that high glucose level is throwing off our osmolality and actually giving us a pseudo-hyponatremia. We really need to correct the glucose and the sodium will correct itself. In a patient who is hyponatremic yet hyperosmolar, the cause of the elevated osmolality must be addressed. Now, the most common cause, by far, is glucose. However, excessive lipids can do this as well, as is the case when it comes to toxicology; heavy alcohols such as methanol, ethylene glycol, isopropyl alcohol, and even ethanol. Most patients we will treat have low serum osmolality. So, if we have a patient with low sodium and low serum osmolality, our next step is to evaluate the patient's volume. Does the patient have normal volume, low volume or high volume?

Here is the story and here is the mnemonic. You have a guy in the Navy who gets on a boat and goes across the sea on a battleship to a port of ill repute. He gets off the boat and visits a brothel. He gets back on the boat and comes back to the United States. Now, the United States government and our CDC is very concerned about our military personnel going overseas where they have different sexually transmitted diseases and bringing them back to the United States. So, the CDC is waiting on the dock and say, "Hey you, you need a VD dart." A VD dart is a venereal disease dart. This is basically a shot a sailor would get in the butt that contains a bunch of prophylactic medications to prevent them from spreading any diseases in the United States. So, the **MNEMONIC** has to do with a U on the ship, which means a patient who is U-volemic, the **MNEMONIC** is **SHIP**.

S	**SYNDROME OF HIGH ANTIDIURETIC**
H	**HYPOTHYROIDISM**
I	**INAPPROPRIATE WATER FOR A CHILD**
P	**PSEUDOHYPONATREMIA**

The **S** stands for syndrome of inappropriate high antidiuretic hormone, **H**-hypothyroidism, **I**-inappropriate feeding of water to a child and **P**-pseudohyponatremia. First, let's look at U-volemic hyponatremia. SIADH or syndrome of inappropriately high antidiuretic hormone is often a diagnosis of exclusion and can be a very tricky diagnosis. This can be caused typically by pulmonary disease, someone who has lung cancer or tuberculosis. That tumor can secrete antidiuretic hormone and cause the patient's volume status to stay normal yet drop their sodium. Hypothyroidism can do this as well when you check a TSH. Inappropriate feeding of water to a child can happen when parents who have relatively low income are trying to save some money by diluting the child's formula. Instead of getting four scoops of formula to water, they will give two scoops of formula to water, and the child really is not getting the electrolytes he needs and getting too much water.

Water intake is an important factor. Psychogenic polydipsia occurs when a patient with mental retardation issues, if left with an unrestricted access to water, can drink 10 to 20 pounds of water per day. Their body will help them pee out the water but will drop their sodium to a really severe level, causing seizures. Hyponatremia is a real problem with ultra endurance athletes where if they are running for hours at a time and not replacing sodium appropriately, this can cause their sodium to drop. There have actually been deaths reported in ultra endurance events because sodium has dropped so low. So, with U-volemic patients, you want to think **SHIP**, syndrome of inappropriate high antidiuretic hormone, hypothyroidism, inappropriate feeding of water to a child, or psychogenic polydipsia. Now, the mnemonic for hypovolemia is **VDDART**.

V	VOMITING
D	DIARRHEA
D	DIURETIC
A	ADDISON'S DISEASE
R	RENAL TUBULAR ACIDOSIS
	(TOXIN/TRAUMA)
T	THIRD SPACING OF FLUID

The first three are really easy. In VDDART, V is vomiting, D is diarrhea, and D is diuretic. Those are easy. A stands for Addison's disease. Addison's disease really means add some cortisol. Addison's disease are patients who have low cortisol states or kind of have acute adrenal insufficiency. The way to fix this is to add some cortisol.

Addison's disease is a really tricky diagnosis and always has been. These people come in with vague symptoms of abdominal pain and low blood pressure, and the diagnosis actually takes **MAGIK** is a mnemonic for the causes of Addison's disease.

M	MENINGITIS
A	ADRENAL HEMMORAGE
G	GRANULOMATOUS DISEASE
I	IMMUNOCOMPROMIZED
K	KETOCONAZOLE (ANITFUNGAL MED)

M is meningitis caused by neisseria meningitis. A is adrenal hemorrhage which may happen from childbirth or trauma. G is granulomatous disease such as sarcoidosis or tuberculosis. I is immunocompromised state such as HIV or chronic steroid use. K is ketoconazole, which is an antifungal medication. Of interest is pheochromocytoma, which is a tumor of the adrenal gland that secretes too much catecholamines or too much epinephrine. Ketoconazole can be used to suppress pheochromocytomas. Going back to the mnemonic of

VDDART where vomiting, diarrhea, diuretics, A is Addison's disease, R is renal tubular acidosis or has to do with an acute trauma or toxin to the kidneys, and T is third spacing of fluids which means fluid weeps out into the interstitium such as seen with burns or pancreatitis.

Hypervolemic patients has to do with a CDC where C stands for cirrhosis, D, well it's not really D, it's actually N for nephrotic syndrome, and the last C stands for congestive heart failure.

When a patient's sodium is off we have to be really concerned about how we correct it. We cannot correct sodium more than 12 millimoles per kilogram over a 24-hour period of time because this can cause pontine demylenationysis, which occurs when there are too-rapid fluid changes in the brain. This can cause brain swelling and death. So, once again when altering someone's sodium, you really cannot go more than 12 millimoles in a 24-hour period or half of a millimole per hour. Treatment of this sodium deficiency really depends on the cause. If someone is hypovolemic with hyponatremia, the treatment is I.V. fluids, where if the patient is hypervolemic and hyponatremic, the treatment is fluid restriction or taking fluid back from them such as with diuretics. We can get ourselves in trouble here, so proceed with caution. If we have a patient whom we think is dehydrated and we are giving them I.V. fluids and they really turn out to be hypervolemic, we can make the sodium worse. We really want to go slow and treat the volume status appropriately.

How can we tell if the patient is hypovolemic or hypervolemic? There are four parts of our history and physical exam that we can use and four lab tests making a total of eight tests. How can we help a patient's volume status? One is by physical exam, checking if they are dry, and also their axilla and their groin. The main way we would do this is to look in their mouth. In a child, do they have spit bubbles and saliva? If so, they are not dehydrated, and the body will just not waste water on the creation of drool. If it looks like the tongue has tacky paint, this suggests someone who may be dehydrated. Next, we would do orthostatic vital signs, which means we would check blood pressure and pulse in the supine, sitting and then standing positions. What you will do is have the patient lie flat for two minutes and let their body kind of equilibrate, then check pulse and blood pressure. Next, you would sit them up, have them wait for two minutes, and recheck pulse and blood pressure. Then, do the same thing standing. Now, typical response would be quick compensation. If someone gets up in the middle of the night to go to the bathroom, their blood pressure and heart rate would remain relatively constant. Someone who is dehydrated or hypovolemic, like someone who just recently gave blood, when they stand up, has a rapid drop of the systolic blood pressure and the heart rate goes up. This suggests hypovolemia and is useful to work up someone who is hypovolemic.

Number three is to get a good history. Document if someone has been having diarrhea or vomiting or in a child's case, you want to see how much fluid they had taken in over the last 12 hours versus how much goes out, such as how many diapers have they gone through or the number of times they have urinated. Number four is urinary output and again, you can get this from history, but from a hospital perspective, this is where it is helpful to place a Foley catheter. Now, when you first place a Foley catheter in a patient you think may be dehydrated, they are going to have 100 to 200 cc of urine in their bladder. This is not what we are interested in. Say you put a Foley catheter in and get 200 cc out; that is irrelevant. That does not suggest dehydration or hydration. What we are concerned about is how much they are making from here on out. A normal adult should make about ½ cc per kg per hour. I am not much into formulas but a good gauge is about 70 cc per two hours. In a patient putting out less than that, you should really be concerned about hypovolemia and/or shock.

When looking at a patient's volume status from lab values, we want to see how the BUN is elevated relative to creatinine. If greater than 20 in the BUN to creatinine ratio, that suggests dehydration. Now, with urine, we are going to look at specific gravity. If the specific gravity is very high suggesting the urine is concentrated, that would indicate the patient is dehydrated. The FeNa, which stands for the fractional excretion of sodium, is helpful. This test basically looks at how much sodium we are urinating out versus how much sodium we are absorbing. Normally the body will pee out only about 1% of our sodium. It is normal physiology of the kidney to retain a lot of the sodium. Someone who is dehydrated will have a low FeNa, so it will be less than 1%. The FeNa is helpful, not as much to determine whether the patient is dehydrated, but more to determine if their elevation in renal functions are from dehydration versus renal disease, which we will talk more about in a later chapter. Lastly is a serum sodium which, again, if the sodium is high, they are dry. If it is low, we need a more detailed.

Next we are going to talk about potassium. Potassium is our main intracellular cation. Potassium is our most important electrolyte. 99% of potassium resides within a cell and is in charge of muscle function, be it our skeletal muscle or our heart. Errors in potassium cause people to die, so, it is a very important electrolyte to have a firm grip on. The number one cause of an elevated potassium level, without any question, is lab error. Now, this does not necessarily mean that the lab did something wrong. It means that the sample most likely was traumatically drawn. The specimen could also have been hemolyzed, which would cause red blood cells to abnormally break down, resulting in an abnormal elevation of potassium. So, the first step always when dealing with hyperkalemia is to validate the data. Ask the lab about their hemolysis of the sample and if that is not completely spelled out, have it redrawn. So, always, always, always think "lab error."

Potassium affects the heart dramatically. When potassium is found to be elevated, we need to make sure the heart is okay, and the bedside test for that is a 12-lead EKG. Now, the EKG criterion for hyperkalemia is easy with the simple mnemonic of thinking of a coat hanger. Now, if we take a coat hanger and bend it out like a QRS complex, so if we have a coat hanger that is bent into a P-wave, a QRS and a T-wave, then we put both ends of the coat hanger in a clamp. Now, we take a pair of pliers and pull up on the T-wave representing the three EKG changes of hyperkalemia where the first step is peaked T-waves. If you keep pulling, hopefully you can picture the QRS complex which will widen. Lastly, the P-wave will flatten. So, the three changes on an EKG of hyperkalemia are peaked T-waves, wide QRS and flat P-waves.

Now, the treatment for hyperkalemia has three different categories. The first is to protect the heart. The second is to shift potassium back into the cell. The third is to remove the potassium from the body. Step 1 – protect the heart. If there is confirmed hyperkalemia and EKG changes, they need calcium. Calcium is cardioprotective for 30-45 minutes, and this can be in the form of calcium gluconate or calcium chloride. Different reference books suggest different formulations of calcium, and it really does not matter which you use. Just know that calcium chloride has a higher concentration at about 3:1 of calcium compared to calcium gluconate. So, if you have EKG changes and hyperkalemia, the first step is calcium. It has been asked of me, "What are the EKG criteria to say that the T-wave is peaked and thus requiring calcium?" My best advice is, if you look at the T-wave and it looks so big that you would not want to sit on it, call it hyperkalemia and treat with calcium. Now, look at the risks versus the benefits. If you are wrong and the patient really did not have hyperkalemia, and you treated them with an amp of calcium, it's really no big deal. It may drop their blood pressure a bit, but overall, calcium is pretty well tolerated I.V. If, on the other hand, you were right and it was indeed hyperkalemia, you potentially could save their life and prevent them from going into a lethal arrhythmia. So, EKG changes and hyperkalemia, treat with calcium.

Next, we want to shift potassium back into the cell. There are three ways to do this, with insulin glucose, sodium bicarbonate or high dose of Proventil. A mechanism I would suggest to you folks is that potassium follows an osmolality load, which means that if glucose changes from in the cell to in the vasculature, potassium is kind of sucked along with it. So, if you give someone glucose and then give them insulin, that insulin is going to cause the glucose to go into the cell. Now, when that glucose goes into the cell, it will take potassium with it. We can use this therapeutically. When someone comes in, is hyperkalemic and are euglycemic (which means their glucose is normal), we give them an amp of dextrose and then right after that, we give them 10 units of insulin. This will cause the potassium to transiently go lower. Now, of concern here, and I know there have been case reports to suggest this, by giving glucose I.V., it means actually giving the patient a transient hyperosmolar state. That transient hyperosmolar state will cause potassium to leave the cell for a small amount of time. If you have a patient who is right on the brink of going into a lethal arrhythmia, this could kick them over the edge. So, I do not recommend this as a first line therapy to treat hyperkalemia.

A second way to shift potassium intra-cellularly is with sodium bicarbonate. From a mechanism's perspective, if you have someone who is in a metabolic acidosis, they are going to have hydrogen ions floating around in the blood vessels. Now, hydrogen is a +1 charge. The body freaks out at this. The body hates this. The body will attempt to normalize pH by pulling hydrogen into the cell. The cell cannot tolerate that so in turn, it is going to kick out a +1 charge so that in a metabolic acidosis, they would have a high hydrogen ion concentration, and the body is going to try and pull that hydrogen into the cell and in turn, kick out a potassium. So, metabolic acidoses are almost always hyperkalemic. They kind of go together. Now, on the opposite side of the coin, if we make someone alkalotic by giving sodium bicarbonate, we reverse this. So, sodium bicarbonate is another alternative to shifting potassium back into the cell. Lastly, high-dose Proventil means giving the patient three and four nebulized treatments all in a row. This will drive potassium into the cell, though the exact mechanism of this is not quite known.

To remove potassium from the body, we have three different mechanisms as well. One is Kayexalate, which can be given in 15 or 30 g. It can be given orally or as a rectal retention enema. This is kind of a binder of potassium. It sucks potassium out of the intestinal tract and you poop it out. It is a really common thing to do, and all providers should be familiar with using Kayexalate. Loop diuretics will also cause the potassium to go lower, yet this should not be used therapeutically. Like, someone with a potassium of 6.3, you should not give them 80 of Lasix in an attempt to drop potassium. It would be better to use the Kayexalate. Lastly, hemodialysis is used in severe cases or in patients who have hyperkalemia primarily from renal failure.

So, in summary, if a patient who comes in for whatever reason, you check their labs and they have a potassium of 6.4, you have two tests that you need to do right away. One is to repeat the lab value and verify the lab value. Have them come back and redraw the sample. The second thing to do is an EKG. If the EKG is normal, you've got some time to wait for the second sample. If the EKG shows signs of hyperkalemia (peaked Ts, wide QRS, or flat P-waves), the patient needs to be treated with calcium. Now, shifting potassium back into the cell is not the best way to treat hyperkalemia. You should use these treatments in conjunction. So, if I gave someone sodium bicarbonate to shift it back into the cell, this may buy me about an hour or two before the potassium weeps back out. It would be best to give bicarbonate with Kayexalate so they can work together. So, as it has moved into the cell, that gives you some time, and they are pooping it out of the body. I recently had a patient who came in to the emergency room with vague symptoms and had a potassium level of 6.7, which we did verify by lab draws. There were no EKG changes, and this patient I actually treated with bicarbonate, insulin glucose and Kayexalate, all three.

Now, we are going to talk about chloride, bicarb and anion gap. The chloride, clinically, is really useless as is the bicarb by itself. The reason why they are of benefit is to calculate an anion gap. The anion gap formula is sodium minus (chloride + bicarb). Now, a normal anion gap is less than 16 or in the pediatric population, age divided by 4+4.

Bicarbonate is made in the kidney. It takes hours to days to actually generate bicarb. Now, when there is a "funky" acid, this will cause the bicarbonate to precipitously drop. It's this low bicarb that gives us an elevated anion gap when you do the math and apply the formula. Now, a positive anion gap is greater than 16. We are not concerned if it is low or normal. We just want to know if it is elevated. Now, a positive anion gap implies a positive "funky" acid. This "funky" acid is any acid that is exogenous to the body that is causing us to be sick. So, a positive anion gap equals a positive "funky" acid, which equals a metabolic acidosis. Once again, a positive anion gap equals positive "funky" acid that we need to find and diagnose which equals a metabolic acidosis. Now, carbon dioxide in the body is an acid. So, under normal circumstances, if you are sitting down reading this book and you decide to take 50 deep breaths in and out, what you will do is blow off carbon dioxide, which is an acid. If you are losing acid, you will make your body become more alkalotic and thus put your body into a respiratory alkalosis.

If you are in a metabolic acidosis, (implied by a positive anion gap and a "funky" acid in the body) your body is going to freak out because it has an acid in the body that it cannot tolerate. The body will compensate from a respiratory perspective by breathing fast. This rapid breathing from a metabolic acidosis is known as **KUSSMAL** breathing. **KUSSMAL**, coincidentally, happens to be the mnemonic for the main causes of a metabolic acidosis where K is ketones, U is uremia, S is sepsis, S is salicylates, M is methanol or other heavy alcohols, A is aldehyde or all others such as iron or isoniazid and L is lactacidosis.

K	**KEYTONES**
U	**UREMIA**
S	**SEPSIS**
S	**SALICYLATES**
M	**METHANOL**
A	**ALDEHYDE**
L	**LACTACIDOSIS**

Talking about those in a little more detail, K in ketones has to do with diabetic ketoacidosis or a starvation ketoacidosis, which could occur in someone who has fasted for a prolonged period of time or even someone who has been on the Adkins diet or low carbohydrate diet. Uremia refers to someone in renal failure with a backup of all their toxins in the body that cannot be properly filtered by the kidneys. S for sepsis has to do with an overwhelming body infection which we talked about work up for under white blood cell count, to include a good temperature, a CBC, blood cultures x2, and a chest x-ray. S is for salicylates, which is an aspirin overdose or a salicylic acid. These patients will have tinnitus (or an abnormal ringing in the ears), and they will appear pretty sick.

When a grandma comes in saying she took some Tylenol for her headache, do not assume that she really knows what she is talking about and it really was Tylenol. If it is an over the counter medication, assume that it could be aspirin and anybody with a metabolic acidosis just check a salicylate level. M is for ethanol or other heavy alcohols, and this could be isopropyl alcohol, methanol, ethanol, any of the heavy alcohols. And, if you recall under sodium, these heavy alcohols will cause a high osmolality. And, if you are working up a patient with hyponatremia, remember that the first step is to check serum osmolality. If the sodium is low and the osmolality is high, a heavy alcohol could be the cause of this. It is from this work up that we would check an osmolar gap, which is really beyond the scope of this text and more for an advanced toxicology class.

Aldehyde is kind of an antiquated chemical but with this, you should think of all others such as iron or isoniazid, isoniazid being a treatment for tuberculosis. It is isoniazid that really drains B6 stores. So, people who are taking INH (or isoniazid) will be on B6 and it so happens that if someone has a bad overdose for INH, the treatment would be B6. L is lactacidosis, which could be found in someone who had prolonged hypoxia to the muscles or could be from Glucophage. Glucophage is in the biguanide class. It works in the liver for diabetes and patients who are on Glucophage are more prone to lactacidosis. There is concern for people on Glucophage who need I.V. contrast studies, and patients who need an I.V. contrast for an angiogram or pulmonary CAT scan to rule out pulmonary embolism. If they are on Glucophage and need a contrast study, the work up is to check renal functions. If these tests are normal, you would go ahead and do the study and hold the Glucophage. Two days later you would recheck renal functions. If they are normal, the patient can restart the Glucophage. If the patient's renal functions are abnormal in the first place such as with a creatinine of 1.8, the study would be held and dye would not be given until the patient was hydrated enough that the creatinine came down to normal.

When we talk about acid base from a basic perspective, we need to talk about a fast response and slow response. The fast response is carbon dioxide or change in the patient's breathing patterns. A patient can alter how they breathe relatively quickly. It is kind of like switching a light switch and having the light bulb turn on quickly. A slow response has to do more with flicking a light switch and it being like an iron that needs a little bit of time to get heated up. Whenever there is an acid base problem, there will be a compensatory response by the body. Metabolic problems refer to problems with bicarbonate where respiratory problems refer to problems with carbon dioxide. A metabolic acidosis, once again in, suggests a positive anion gap, a "funky" acid that we need to find, and **KUSSMAL** breathing which is a hyperventilatory breathing in an attempt to blow off carbon dioxide. We must first get a good history, then find the acid, check a ketone level, check renal functions, do a septic work up, check a salicylate level, and then look for a heavy alcohol, either by serum osmolality or an osmolar gap. Then, see if the patient has taken iron, isoniazid and/or check a lactic acid level. The KUSSMAL breathing from a metabolic acidosis is referred to as a respiratory compensation for the metabolic acidosis. We will talk about acid base in greater detail in a later chapter.

Renal functions refer to BUN and creatinine. Now, do not make the mistake of calling the BUN a "bun." That is a rookie mistake. It is referred to a BUN meaning blood urea nitrogen. Now, if elevated, that is referred to as azotemia. Another renal function is known as the creatinine. Now, creatinine is a breakdown product of muscle and stays relatively constant. A normal reference value for creatinine is less than 1.5, but that is quite variable based on the muscle mass of the individual. If you have a frail 90-year-old lady who weighs 80 lbs and her creatinine is 1.5, that demonstrates significant renal insufficiency. However, when a body builder with a large muscles has a creatinine of 1.7, that may be a completely normal value for this larger gentleman.

If renal functions are elevated, we need to figure out if it is renal, prerenal or postrenal. We must identify this. Prerenal problems have to do with the blood flow going into the kidneys. This is either dehydration or congestive heart failure. Both of these states mean the body is not getting adequate blood flow to the kidneys to keep the renal functions adequate. A way to tell if this is a prerenal problem is to look at the BUN to creatinine ratio. If the ratio is greater than 20, it suggests a prerenal problem. A renal cause of azotemia means that the kidneys are actually diseased and sick. A way to help with this is your BUN and creatinine ratio. Again, if less than 20, that suggests a sick kidney. This is also a time when that fractional excretion of sodium or FeNa is helpful because a FeNa greater than 2 says that the body is not filtering sodium the way it should and again implies a sick kidney.

The most common postrenal problem, by far, is the prostate. Do a rectal exam and see if the prostate is enlarged. Talk to the patient about the history of urinary flow. Is it easy to initiate flow? Do they feel like they empty their bladder completely? The prostate is kind of like a doughnut that the urethra goes through, and when the prostate becomes enlarged, it pinches down on the urethra. A patient who has an enlarged prostate, will void, yet not completely empty their bladder because of the pressure on their urethra. So, you would ask them, "Do you feel like you are completely emptying your bladder after you pee?" If a patient has elevated BUN or creatinine, you need to look at the BUN to creatinine ratio and apply that to patient care. Students can often get confused here. If you have a ratio that is greater than 20 yet the BUN to creatinine values are in normal range, we do not care about that. We do not look at ratio if the BUN to creatinine are normal. So, once again we only look at the BUN to creatinine ratio if the functions are elevated.

CHAPTER 3

ANTIBIOTICS and MICROBIOLOGY

How do we diagnose an infection? I think it is important to remember that common things happen commonly. If it walks like a duck and quacks like a duck, guess what? It's a duck. If someone comes in with fever, sore throat and yucky looking tonsils, 99 out of 100 times it is going to be strep pharyngitis. As you become experienced in medicine, when you see someone with a sore throat and fever, and you examine the throat, and one side of the tonsils is big and swollen, and the uvula is pushed over to the side, you realize this does not look like a normal strep throat. You have to take more appropriate steps to diagnose or get someone smarter than you involved.

So, how do we diagnose a specific bug to target for antibiotic selection? Well, empirical therapy really is our best guess. Next are cultures: blood, urine, sputum, cerebrospinal fluid or stool. The problem with the culture is that it takes 1-2 days to come back, and a patient who is truly bacteremic or septic would succumb to their infection if we did not treat sooner. The culture that is indeed positive is helpful to target antibiotic therapy, 1-2 days out, when it becomes available. Antigen testing is very specific. Serology testing to a specific germ such is legionella or lyme disease is not commonly used. A gram stain could be used of any secretion we can get, be it sputum, lumbar puncture or joint aspirate. We can send that to the lab acutely and have them do a gram stain and see if we can't highlight whether this is a gram-negative germ or a gram-positive germ. The shape and color can give us an idea of what germ it is. Similar to the antigen testing, as much as it is an option, it is rarely employed.

What is the worst thing that could happen when writing an antibiotic prescription? First off, if you write a prescription for someone who is allergic and they have a severe reaction to it, it is very difficult to defend medically or legally. When a patient says, "I have an allergy to penicillin," you want to document the reaction. If they say, "My belly becomes upset," it is not truly an allergic reaction but more of a side effect of the medication. Allergic reactions that we would be concerned about are rash, itching, hives, and swollen throat. Those are the kind of reactions that are considered life threatening, and would be gross malpractice to give someone a medication that they are allergic to.

Do not give antibiotics such as fluoroquinolne to a pregnant woman. That could be harmful to the baby or harmful to mom. Every woman of childbearing age be assumed pregnant until proven otherwise. So, if a 24-year-old woman comes in with a kidney stone and a urinary tract infection, it would be negligent to put her on fluoroquinolone without checking a pregnancy test first. Also, be cautious when prescribing antibiotics to women on birth control pills. Birth control pills are absorbed through the intestines via bowel flora which means that the germs in a woman's gut allows the birth control pills to be absorbed. If you put a woman who is on birth control pills on antibiotics, that is going to kill or stun the bowel flora, therefore the birth control pills will not be absorbed. If you put someone who is on birth control pills on an antibiotic, you have to warn them to have protected intercourse for at least 30 days.

Missing a more important infection is another serious consequence of prescribing antibiotics. A child could come in with a fever and be diagnosed with an ear infection, when the actual pathology is pneumonia. So, you musts look for the most severe infection and treat accordingly. Lastly, you could prescribe the wrong antibiotic. That means you just do not know the spectrum of antibiotic coverage well enough and prescribe an antibiotic that is not effective for that particular infection such as prescribing penicillin for a cellulitis.

You always have to ask yourself, "Could this be viral, and is it appropriate to prescribe antibiotics? Do we need an amoxacebo?" I found early in my career when I was less confident in patient care that I wrote a lot of antibiotic prescriptions for patients I was relatively sure had a virus. Now, why would I do something like that? I personally felt it had to do with patient expectations. A constant theme throughout this book is that I will ask you, "What is good medicine? And, what determines if you practice good medicine on any given day, on any given patient encounter?" I would suggest that good medicine is based on the expectation of the patient, and if the patient left feeling like you did a good job, then you did do a good job. And, I would suggest that if the patient left and did not feel like they were well cared for, then for that particular patient, you did not practice good medicine. It is kind of like going to a restaurant and ordering a meal. The food could be tremendous, it could be wonderful, but if the waitress was not good or was not attentive or if you felt the waitress was rude, you would leave with negative feelings about that particular restaurant.

I feel it is the same thing with medicine. It is a service industry. So when mom brings her kid in at 2 in the morning, fearful that this child's infection could be life threatening, when you as a provider look at them and say, "This is just a virus," our job is now to educate mom that this is not a severe infection or a life-threatening infection. Now, if mom is insistent on an antibiotic, do we prescribe it? I would suggest that you always want to practice medicine to your best integrity, but do not back yourself into a hole by saying, "This is only a virus, and I am not going to prescribe antibiotics," because you will have parents leave upset and then bad things come back to haunt you.

I remember early in my career I had a young child come in with parents who were concerned as the child had a fever, diarrhea and was a little fussy. I examined the child and diagnosed a virus stating that he would be okay. The next day, my boss pulled me into his office stating that the child left the ER and went to another hospital where he was diagnosed with pneumonia. My boss just wanted me to be aware that the chart was going to be pulled for review. I was extremely upset about this thinking that I missed a bacterial pneumonia in a child. I actually went out of my way to call the other hospital and had a copy of the chart sent to me. When I got a copy of the chart, it became clear that the emergency room provider at the other hospital only ordered a basic chemistry and a chest x-ray. He did not order a CBC. The official report on the chest x-ray was that it was normal. With that said, my boss quickly dismissed this case from peer review. This told me that the parent went there with the expectation of receiving an antibiotic and implied to the provider there that they were mistreated at the hospital that I was at, thus prompting the provider to call it pneumonia and treat with antibiotics even though there were no objective findings of that.

There is indeed an increasing antibiotic resistance problem throughout the world, and I feel that every time we prescribe an antibiotic that is not necessary, we contribute to that. Understanding that it is important to have satisfied patients within reason, it is also important to practice good medicine. I subscribe more to the philosophy of educate, not medicate. Now, when I have a child whose parent I feel is insistent on nudging an antibiotic, I do go out of my way to educate and say, "There is no way I can know for sure whether this is truly an infection that will respond to antibiotics. I don't think so." I always tell them, "Based on what I am seeing here, I would not put my child on antibiotics right now." I would then go on to say, "The chances of your child getting better in a day or two are very high." A technique I have employed is called the delayed antibiotic prescription which basically means that I do write them a prescription, but I tell the parent, "Listen, you are coming into the emergency room today and I would sure hate for you to come back twice for the same thing. I am confident your child has a virus, and if we put him on an antibiotic, he is going to get better in a day or two. If you go home and use Tylenol, Motrin and fluids, he will get better in a day or two." What I do is empower them with the prescription saying, "If you feel your child really needs antibiotic, you can go ahead and start him on it. Or, if you want to wait a day and see if he turns the corner, then you can start him on it." I feel this has the patients leave satisfied. You are not completely giving in to writing useless prescriptions, and to the best of my knowledge, about 50% of these prescriptions do indeed get filled. But, I do feel it is a happy medium between keeping patients happy and practicing good medicine.

Let's move on to microbiology. There are four general classes of germs. We have gram positives, gram negatives, anaerobes and atypicals. We are not going to be as concerned about viruses, fungals or parasites. Let's start out talking about the six, gram positive bugs that we need to be concerned with. Two begin with the letter S, two begin with the letter C, and we have a D and an L. The two that begin with S are staph and strep. Staphylococcus is primarily a skin infection, which lives on the skin and lives in moist areas such as axilla, groin and nares. It produces beta-lactamase, which basically means it is penicillin resistant. Now, staphylococcus lives on the skin and has lived on our skin since the dawn of man. Penicillin is made from mold. Mold has also lived on our skin since the dawn of man. Any time you have an organism that ingests something chronically, they are going to become resistant to it. Therefore, all staph is resistant to penicillin. You will hear about MRSA or ORSA. MRSA is methicillin resistant staph aureus and ORSA is oxacillin resistant staph aureus. Methicillin and oxacillin are both penicillins that were specifically made to kill staph. Well, staph has become smarter and more resistant. So, if you get a strain of MRSA, this is a very stubborn strain of staph. These patients are atypically isolated in the hospital and therefore patient contact needs to be made with gloves, gown and mask. There are a couple different strep. The first is pyogenes, which actually means "pus-producing." It is strep pyogenes that causes strep throat and these patients present with fevers, headache and sore throat. Strep throat does not give upper respiratory infection type symptoms like sniffles or cough. Those are not consistent with strep. Strep is strictly like a red-hot poker on the back of the throat with sore throat, fever and headache. Now, when you look into the throat, you can see exudate on the tonsils, you can see red, beefy tonsils. It actually has a very distinct smell that you will learn over the years treating strep throat.

Medically, there can be a complication of strep throat where the strep actually enters the blood stream and seats itself on the heart valves and can give the patient valvular heart disease. This is indeed antibiotic related meaning that as we discovered penicillin in the 40s and really starting aggressively treating strep throat, the incidents of rheumatic fever has dramatically decreased. You will have patients with history of rheumatic fever as a child, but these are typically elderly folks. Post-streptococcal glomerulonephritis is an insult to the kidneys that occurs after a strep throat. This can give the patients a kind of tea-colored urine and a degree of azotemia. Post-streptococcal glomerulonephritis is not antibiotic related. This is not related to whether the patient had antibiotics or not. It is just something that kind of happens from time to time in people with strep throat. Usually it is self-limiting.

When patients hear the term scarlet fever they get kind of scared as they remember hearing horror stories about scarlet fever. Scarlet fever really means that they have strep throat and a sandpaper rash. There is just a toxin that is produced by this particular strep that gives a rash. You need to explain to your patients that it is no big deal, just means that there is strep throat and a rash. Treatment is no different.

Strep viridans is basically a strep that lives in the mouth. It can cause endocarditis from dental work. If a patient has a degree of valvular heart disease already, and needs to get dental work, we will put them on prophylactic antibiotics to protect from strep viridans.

Strep enterococcus is a germ that resides in the gastrointestinal tract (thus the term entero). It can be seen in urinary tract infections and is extremely resistant to all the cephalosporins. You will hear the term VRE or Vancomycin resistant enterococcus. It is similar to MRSA or ORSA. This particular germ is very resistant to our potent antibiotic Vancomycin, therefore patients with strep enterococcus require isolation. As a note, MRSA, ORSA and VRE, though stubborn bugs to kill, are not more virulent. If I go into a room where the patient has MRSA, it does not mean this is going to be an aggressive staph infection that is going to eat away at my skin. It just means that I may become contaminated with it and spread it to someone else. Strep pneumococcus is a critically important germ to know because we will see this time and time again for the rest of our careers. It does cause bad things to happen. It has a very distinct gram shape, which is a gram positive diplococci (gram negative diplococci refers to neisseria). There are 84 capsules to strep pneumococcus, and once a patient gets infected with one, the body will produce antibodies so you can never get it again. So, in theory we can really only get strep pneumococcus 84 times. This germ is primarily responsible for pneumonia and meningitis in adults, and otitis media in children.

It is from this very infectious strep pneumococcus germ that we have developed the Pneumovax, which is a pneumococcal vaccine. The Pneumovax encompasses 25 of the most common capsular antigens, which means we are getting 25 out of the 84. This immunizes the patient to the most common forms of strep pneumococcus. I have had it asked of me, "Well, why don't we have all 84 in there?" and I just don't know. Patients who really need to Pneumovax are patients without a spleen. These are people who have had trauma in the past and had their spleen removed or people who have sickle cell anemia whose spleens are basically not functioning because the sickling of the cells has fried their spleen over time. Also, people over 65 years of age, patients with multiple medical problems or patients who are immunocompromised must have the Pneumovax.

Clostridium is a gram positive spore-forming germ responsible for four clinically relevant infections we need to be aware of. Clostridium botulium is basically a disease of paralysis of the muscles. This is where we would not give honey to children less than one year of age, although the incidence of this happening is quite rare and happened in a small outbreak in California. In my clinical career, we did have a lady who presented to the emergency room with dysphagia which we thought was from a benzodiazepine overdose, or a stroke. In CAT scanning, she decompensated and went into respiratory arrest and ended up intubated. Over the next couple of days, she did not respond normally, and in the process of this, it was realized that she could move her big toe on command. From tests that were sent to our main laboratory, it was found that she did indeed have botulism from some poorly prepared fish.

The next genus of clostridium is tetani. This is where we give the tetanus shot. Now, you should be updated with the tetanus shot every 10 years or every 5 years with high-risk or tetanus-prone wounds. A buzzword for tetanus is trismus. This is lock jaw or that locked appearance with spasm of the muscles in the jaw that occur when people have tetanus. If a patient has never been immunized and needs antibodies to tetanus, we would give them immunoglobulin. Most people in the United States have had their regular shots, and therefore a tetanus-prone wound only requires the tetanus shot. If you have a patient who has never been immunized, as is common in the

Amish community where I work, and they have a tetanus-prone wound, not only would we give them the tetanus shot but would give the immunoglobulin as well. As a side note, when this is ordered, it is ordered as dT 0.5mg IM.

Clostridium perfringens causes gas gangrene. This can be of an extremity, usually in diabetics. When we do an x-ray of a limb that we think may have gas gangrene in it, we are actually looking for black streaks of air within the muscle.

The next clostridium species is known as difficile, also known as pseudomembranous colitis. This is an infection of the bowel wall of the large intestine, typically antibiotic related. So, when any patient comes in with diarrhea, one of the big questions you want to ask is whether they were recently on antibiotics. A buzz word for antibiotic-related pseudomembranous colitis is Clindamycin. There is a really high incidence of pseudomembranous colitis based on the text books. Treatment is either Vancomycin or Flagyl. The way to think about Vancomycin is a van with a big plus on the side of it, like an ambulance. Flagyl is used for anaerobic infections.

Our fourth germ is called Corynebacterium. This causes diphtheria. It causes kind of a pseudomembrane in the throat that is really not seen anymore because of the vaccinations. The next gram positive germ is called listeria. This can cause neonatal meningitis or can cause food poisoning in adults.

The last gram positive germ is called bacillus. This is responsible for the anthrax outbreak. I was actually in Desert Storm and penetrated into Kuwait with the US Marine Corps back in 1991. When we went through the ground war, we were actually given pills to take. There are two different pills that we took on different regimines. Now, after the war I actually went to the VA and went through my records, and there was no record of us taking pills. I went through my Senator who got in contact with the Pentagon and reported back that one of the medications we had taken was Cipro to prophylax against bacillus, because of concern that the Iraqi army could use anthrax as a biological agent.

Next, I want to talk about gram negative germs. I want to focus on some of the more important ones, so when you hear the name of a germ, you want to know whether it is a gram positive or an atypical germ. If not one of those, you can make a safe bet that it is a gram negative. The first is neisseria. This causes meningitis, also known as meningococcus. This occurs when people live in close contact, such as students in dorms or military recruits living in close proximity. You must treat all close contacts prophylactically with Rifampin. Rifampin is an antibiotic that causes body secretions, such as tears, sweat and urine, to turn red. On the same note, Pyridium is a pain medication and antispasmodic medication for urinary tract infections. This also turns body fluids red, and you really need to warn patients about this because if you have someone with a urinary tract infection, you put them on Pyridium and all of a sudden their urine turns red, they are going to be coming back to thinking that they now have blood in their urine. Neisseria is a gram negative diplococci. It is important as a clinician for you to know that gram positive diplococci is pneumococcus. Gram negative diplococci is meningococcus. E. Coli, also known as Escherichia, is a gram negative rod. It is the most common germ seen in urinary tract infections, also common in the stool.

Haemophilus influenzae (Latin for blood-loving) also known as H. flu, is the strep pneumo of smokers with pneumonia. It was once thought that H flu was a virus, which is why they named it influenzae even though we now know it is a gram negative. This basically means that when it comes to pneumonia, strep pneumo is the most common germ, but not in smokers. H. flu also causes epiglottis which we really do not see much anymore because of the HIB vaccine, (haemophilus influenzae type B). That caused the epiglottis to become inflamed and causes death in children because it obstructs the airway. This has been pretty much eradicated because of the HIB vaccine. Haemophilus influenzae is a common germ seen in otitis media and also pneumonia. The spirochetes is called that because of its corkscrew like shape. Treponema pallidum causes syphilis where Borrelia Burgdorferi causes lyme disease.

Next is microbacterium which causes tuberculosis. For these patients we would do a PPD, (purified protein derivative) a subcutaneous injection on the arm that health providers need yearly. If the PPD test is positive, meaning there is a localized inflammation at the site of the injection, patients would then go on to get a chest x-ray to make sure there are not pulmonary lesions and that this is not a respiratory infectious risk. As long as it is not, these patients will go on 6-12 months of isoniazid therapy as well as B6. An acid-fast stain is what is required to diagnose by stain. Now, anergy testing is what we do when we have a patient who is immunocompromised such as with HIV, and we need to test for tuberculosis. What we do is injections into the skin of germs that we know a patient has been exposed to in their life such as mumps or candidia. Now, if we inject the skin with mumps candidia and there is an appropriate immune response at the site, we know they have a good enough immune system to respond to the PPD. If we inject the patient with mumps and candidia, and there is no response there and no response to the PPD, we cannot consider the PPD valid.

Number six is klebsiella. This has a tendency to cause pneumonia in alcoholics, so that is kind of a buzzword for alcoholics. Next is pseudomonas. This is just a bad germ and is very stubborn to treat. A lot of times we see this in postoperative wounds. Pseudomonas is always a fun thing to have the operator page overhead in a big hospital. " Paging Dr. Dimonas, Dr. Sue Dimonas." Just a bit of medical humor for you.

Anaerobes are collections of germs that live in places in the body where there is no oxygen such as in abscesses, gallbladder, appendix, diverticulitis, pelvic inflammatory disease or diabetic foot. These are bugs in the gastrointestinal tract, therefore any infection that must originate from the gastrointestinal tract, you really need to be concerned with anaerobic coverage. If we are going to specifically treat someone for anaerobes, two antibiotics need to come to mind. One is Flagyl, or metronidazole, and the other is clindamycin. Some notes about Flagyl, or metronidazole, these people get an Antabuse-like reaction, which means that if they take Flagyl and drink alcohol, this very well could put them into an episode where they throw up. So, we want to tell people on Flagyl to avoid alcohol. Clindamycin is a great antibiotic for gram-positive germs and works wonderfully in patients who have an allergy to penicillin. This also is the antibiotic, as stated before, that is most often indicated with clostridium difficile.

Atypicals are germs that are about the size of viruses yet we can kill them with antibiotics. There are three main players in the atypical class: Mycoplasma, legionella and chlamydia. Mycoplasma is the germ indicated in "walking pneumonia." These are people who have an upper respiratory infection and are not so sick that they cannot go to work but sick enough that they still feel pretty crummy. It can be mistaken for a viral infection, but normally drags itself on for 5, 6, 7, 8, 9 days. The diagnostic test of choice is called cold agglutination antibodies, which can be sent off to the lab. I have read about a bedside test where you take a tube of uncoagulated blood and put it in some ice, and if the red blood cell clumps together, you can safely make the diagnosis of mycoplasma.

Legionella was named from a diagnosis in 1976 where there was an outbreak in a legionnaire's post. Multiple people died from this infection because we did not really know what it was. To test for this, there is a legionella antigen panel. Now, if a patient comes in and has pneumonia, we really need to be concerned that they have this because it is a scary infection once it seats itself. So, any patient who comes in with pneumonia, we are going to treat for atypical infections.

Lastly is chlamydia psittacosis. This is an infection from bird droppings. Chlamydia can also cause a sexually transmitted disease in males and in females. I recall having a patient come in to the emergency room, sent in by a family practice doctor. He was a 17-year-old kid, but big at approximately 220 lbs. The doctor said he looked like he had pneumonia and looked pretty bad in the office and wanted emergency room work up. When he walked in, he looked sick. He was pale and sweaty, and I remember watching him walk through the room. When I evaluated him, his vital signs looked remarkably good. He had a low-grade temperature. He was not hypoxic. His physical exam revealed a lot of symptoms in the right lung, and I really felt this young man had right sided pneumonia. But, when the x-ray came back and his labs came back, his labs showed a relatively normal CBC but he was found to have an infection in his left lung. I remember thinking that this just did not make sense from clinical exam. Everything about this screamed right sided, when his x-ray showed left sided. Again, when we talk about infections, if it walks like a duck and talks like a duck, it is a duck. But, when something is weird, that is when we need to get someone smarter than us involved. So, basically I had his doctor come see the patient thinking this just does not look like a typical bacterial infection. After a prolonged history, it was found that these people did recently have a parrot that died, and was determined that this was an atypical pneumonia caused by chlamydia.

If we are going to treat any patient for an atypical infection, we need to use a macrolide, a ketech or a fluoroquinolone. Now, macrolides have three in the class: Zithromax, erythromycin and Biaxin. Ketech is an upper respiratory antibiotic in its own unique class. Fluoroquinolones is a great antibiotic to treat multiple different infections, which we will talk about more, at a later time.

There are three different general classes of antibiotics that are commonly used that we need to be familiar with. These different classes have different spectrums of coverage. We need to be mostly concerned with whether it covers strep, staph and gram negative germs. These fall in the classifications of penicillins, beta-lactamase penicillins and aminopenicillins.

Basic penicillin covers strep well. If someone has a strep throat or strep pneumococcus pneumonia or strep pneumococcus meningitis, then we can confirm that penicillin is a fine antibiotic and still works well. Penicillin, once again, does not cover staph. Remember that staph is a common germ on the skin, and penicillin comes from mold, so staph chews up and spits out penicillin. So, if someone comes in with a leg cellulitis and we assume it is staph, putting him on penicillin is not a wise choice. Penicillin also does not cover gram negatives.

Beta-lactamase penicillins such as dicloxacillin or nafcillin or oxacillin were specifically made to kill staph, so, when we look at spectrum of coverage and we ask whether it covers strep, yes it does. Does it cover staph? Yes it does. But, it does not cover gram negatives. So, it is the beta-lactamase penicillin that is a strong choice for cellulitis. It is not such a good choice for something like an otitis media where gram negatives are typically involved as a culprit. The p.o. formulation of beta-lactamase penicillin is dicloxacillin. The I.V. formulation is methicillin, nafcillin and oxacillin. Once again, it is a great drug for staph.

The aminopenicillins such as ampicillin or Amoxicillin were made to cover the basic strep molecule and gram negatives, but not staph. So, when we look at the spectrum, yes it covers strep, no it does not cover staph, but yes it does cover gram negatives. Some terms that you may be familiar with or hear… you may have a combination of "ampingent," which stands for ampicillin and gentamycin. Again, ampicillin is strong for strep and for gram negatives. Gentamycin is a strong antibiotic used for gram-negative germs and pseudomonas.

We can use beta-lactamase inhibitors with the aminopenicillins to cover staph. If we want to extend the spectrum of ampicillin or Amoxicillin, we can add a component to the aminopenicillins and thus give beta-lactamase coverage. Augmentin is a combination of Amoxicillin and clavulanic acid. Unasyn is a combination of ampicillin and sulbactam. Zosyn is a combination of piperacillin and tazobactam.

As a general rule, cephalosporins provide very good staph coverage. We talk about cephalosporins in terms of first generation, second generation and third generation. It is important to have a basic understanding of spectrums, and after that it is important to know really two or three cephalosporins. First generation cephalosporins are very good gram positive coverers. They cover staph and strep well, but not so much gram negatives. What you need to know here is Keflex and Ancef. Keflex, pound for pound, is the most common antibiotic I prescribe for skin infections. The I.V. formulation is Ancef, and what will happen is someone will come in with a pretty serious cellulitis that you assume is from a gram positive germ. Either the emergency room or the office practice will give either an I.V. or I.M. dose of Ancef and then start them on Keflex. Second generation cephalosporins really cover all three spectrums pretty well: staph, strep and gram negatives. It is a great intermediary between covering the negatives and positives.

Third generation cephalosporins cover strep well, staph not so well, but cover gram negatives really well. The quintessential third generation cephalosporin is Rocephin. This is a really strong antibiotic for life-threatening infections. As a matter of fact, this is a poop-hits-the-fan kind of antibiotic. If you have someone who comes in looking toxically sick, whether it is a child or an adult, and they have you scared, you can always load them with Rocephin, and it, 19 out of 20 times will cover your most serious, life-threatening germs.

There is a lot of conversation about the allergic reaction to penicillin and the cross reactivity to cephalosporins. So, if someone is allergic to penicillin (meaning they broke out in hives and a rash) what are the chances that they will have that same reaction to cephalosporins? The text books quote 10% cross coverage, so they are saying that if 10 people have an allergic reaction to penicillin, 1 out of the 10 will have that same allergic reaction to cephalosporins. It has been proven clinically that this is not the case, and it is much more like 1%. That is now what experts are saying. Clinically, I can say I have never had a problem using cephalosporins in someone who said they were penicillin allergic. I did a lot of in-patient medication where I would see someone through the emergency department, admit them for pneumonia, and we would cover them with Rocephin and Zithromax, and not once in my career have I had someone who was penicillin allergic have that cross reactivity to the cephalosporins. I am aware it is there, but I think the risk is small. What I will do is question the patient about the reaction. If they had a life-threatening reaction where their throat closed up and they needed epinephrine to open it up, I would not even take that small risk. But, if they said they had a rash or had an upset stomach (which really is not an allergic reaction), or they do not know what happened as a child, I have no problem rolling the dice and using cephalosporins. And, I do feel that is within the standard of care.

Macrolides are good antibiotics to cover atypicals, gram positives and gram negatives. The three that I want to talk about are erythromycin, Zithromax and Biaxin. Erythromycin is kind of the first generation antibiotic in this class and can create a lot of gastrointestinal upset. So, patients will come in saying they are allergic to erythromycin, but when you get a good history, you realize it just made their belly upset, which is quite common side effect. It is good for gram positive germs, and in review, that is staph and strep most commonly, and atypicals. Once again, the atypicals are mycoplasma, legionella and chlamydia. Zithromax has some gram positive and negative coverage plus it does cover atypicals. Zithromax has a long half-life of about 75 hours, so a 3-5 day course stays in a patient for approximately two weeks. My concern about Zithromax is that it just is not a very good antibiotic in someone who really needs antibiotics to get better. If you read the package insert from Zithromax and the PDR, Pfizer will come right out and say it is not a good antibiotic in people with moderate to severe infections and should be used in conjunction with someone who is coming into the hospital to be admitted.

Now, it has been my experience that who gets admitted for pneumonia varies from provider to provider. There are some set standards to say a person with pneumonia needs to be admitted, clear-cut cases, such as an elderly patient who has multiple medical problems and is hypoxic. Without question, this person needs to be admitted. But, what about the young college student with an 02 saturation of 92% and a fever of 103-104°? Is this someone who needs to come into the hospital or could they be loaded with antibiotics in the emergency room and seen by their primary care physician the following day? The package insert from Zithromax says that if they are sick enough to be in the hospital, you should not use Zithromax alone. Biaxin does cover gram positive, gram negatives plus atypicals, and I believe it is the best macrolide.

Bactrim or trimethoprim sulfamethoxazole (TMP SMZ) is a sulfa antibiotic and is used as a first line antibiotic for urinary tract infections. It is very inexpensive and is still effective. This is also used prophylactically for pneumoocystis *chorinine* pneumonia (PCP). Some points about spectrum coverage of Bactrim include studies not showing high resistance to E. Coli and urinary tract infections. What will happen is someone will come in with a urinary tract infection, we will put them on Bactrim, and two days later we will get the culture and sensitivity report showing Bactrim does not cover E. Coli and is resistant to this particular infection. We will call the patient at home, and they will say they are better.

With culture and sensitivities, don't miss the forest for the trees. The tree in front of you is the fact that you have a resistance pattern on your sensitivity. The forest is whether the patient did get better. Now, resistance patterns are a laboratory value. Some lab technician decided that if the mean inhibitory concentration on a Petrie plate is so many millimeters, this is sensitive. If it is so many, it is intermediate. And, if it is so many, it is resistant. So, just because a laboratory value says an antibiotic is resistant to a particular germ does not mean clinically the patient will respond that way. Bactrim is highly concentrated in the urine, and when people urinate it out, they get a high concentration of the Bactrim, and I do not feel that is taken into consideration when they look at the Petrie plate. So, you will read a lot about resistance patterns to Bactrim in 10-20%, but clinically I do not feel it falls into that range. Bactrim is also a deadly combination to use with Coumadin. So, any patient on Coumadin is never placed on Bactrim. I have heard it said that if you want to make someone's INR go as high as it can go, as fast as it can go, place them on a couple doses of Bactrim. I have admitted patients to the hospital with extremely high INRs because someone in a nursing home saw that a patient had a urinary tract infection and blindly put them on Bactrim without checking to see if they were on Coumadin.

The aminoglycosides (Gentamycin) is a big gun antibiotic versus gram negatives, it covers pseudomonas and is also "dirt" cheap. It has really kind of fallen out of favor because of some of the toxicities associated with Gentamycin. They have found that patients who use Gentamycin over an extended length of time have a tendency to have renal disease. This is dose-related and time-use related. Gentamycin also has a problem with ear issues or ototoxicity or 8th cranial nerve toxicity. This does not appear to be dose-related, just appears to be one of those reactions that happens with the use of Gentamycin. I have cared for patients who really had a difficult time hearing, and they said it was because when they were younger they were given some antibiotic (gentamycin) and now don't hear so well.

The aminopenicillins are a good antibiotic if fighting a life-threatening gram negative infection such as E. Coli or pseudomonas. The normal dose used to be about 60-80 mg three times per day, and that is what the older nurses are used to using. Now, we use to 5-8 mg per kg once per day and adjust how much based on their gent level in about 10-16 hours post-dose. So, this basically gives the patients about a dose of 500 mg all at once. This has a tendency to freak out older nurses who call you asking whether you are sure you want this much, because they were scared to death in nursing school about the toxicities and to see that dose makes them think you do not know what you are doing. Overall, though, this antibiotic has fallen out of favor and has been replaced by other forms of gram negative coverage. If someone comes in appearing toxically sick, especially from urinary tract infections, where their blood pressure is borderline, I find that it is in the patient's best interest to give them a one-time dose of gentamycin and cover them with another antibiotic.

We are now going to talk about the fluoroquinolones such as Levaquin, Tequin and Cipro. Overall, this is a very good class of antibiotics. It covers a lot of different germs and a lot of severe infections. It covers gram negatives, gram positives and atypicals. The most common used are Levaquin and Cipro. Levaquin is a very good antibiotic for everything. If you find that you are not very good at microbiology or prescribing antibiotics, and you are thrown into a situation where you have to start seeing patients with infectious diseases, put them all on Levaquin because it will cover everything. It will cover otitis, pneumonia, pharyngitis, appendicitis and diabetic foot ulcers.

I feel that it is an abused antibiotic and should be reserved for people whose spectrum really deems it necessary. It is a very good antibiotic for urinary tract infections. It is a very good antibiotic for gonorrhea. I like to call Levaquin the amiodarone of antibiotics, where amiodarone is a cardiac medication for cardiac arrhythmias, and from an emergency perspective, we can use amiodarone pretty much for anything and be right. It is the same thing with Levaquin. If we use it, we will cover the right germ. My concern is that it is being overused, and there are resistance patterns being seen with strep pneumo.

Cipro is a good antibiotic for gram negatives, for urinary tract infections. It does not cover staph or strep well. So, Cipro would be a very poor choice for a skin infection or pneumonia.

Lets talk about sepsis and what makes a patient septic versus bacteremic. Sepsis is defined as SIRS. This is systemic inflammatory response syndrome. You need two or more of the following which is really pretty easy to qualify for plus a documented infection: A temperature of greater than 102° or less than 96°, a pulse greater than 90, a respiratory rate greater than 20 and lab values demonstrating a white blood cell count of greater than 12, less than 4 or greater than 10 bands. So, once again SIRS is with a temperature, a fast heart rate, a fast respiratory rate a high or low white count or a high band count. Now, this really is clinically easy to qualify for if you look at the definition as set by the Society of Critical Care Providers. If you go by this definition, someone comes in with strep throat and have a fever, are they septic. So, sure they have a documented infection, their pulse is up at 120 because of their fever, and they have a white count of 18,000, so are they truly septic. And, by definition, yes they are, but that is clinically not how we would use the term septic. Septic is a term reserved for someone who has a life-threatening infection.

Septic can further be classified into severe sepsis, septic shock or MODS. Where, severe sepsis is sepsis with organ dysfunction such as hypotension or hypoperfusion or a shock-like state, where lactic acid is produced and urinary output is dropping off, typically less than 70 cc per two hours with or without mental status changes. That kind of denotes someone with severe sepsis. So, an example of this would be the elderly demented lady from the nursing home who is demented at baseline but comes in with a blood pressure systolically of 80 where normally her systolic pressure is 120-130, you bring her in, her heart is racing, she has a fever of 104°, and when you catheterize her, her urine almost looks like pus. That is a patient who qualifies for severe sepsis and we would be aggressive on antibiotic therapy and I.V. fluids.

Septic shock is sepsis that is hypotensive and will not correct itself with I.V. fluids. The lady I spoke about above was loaded with fluids, but it did not make her blood pressure better. These are patients that need I.V. vasopressors, such as dopamine.

MODS stands for multiorgan dysfunction syndrome. This is a person who is at any stage of sepsis, and their body is just shutting down. This is typically considered a near-death situation.

Critically important to any new provider is how we can tell whether we have a sick kid. How can we tell whether a child who comes in with a fever of 102° is someone who just has an otitis media or viral syndrome, of if they have bacterial pneumonia, bacterial meningitis and truly is sick? In my years of experience, it comes down to "the look." How does this child look? Any time you approach a child with a fever, you have to stand there and look at them for 5-10 seconds, and you can get a tremendous amount of information for this. Have the parents take the child's shirt off and just look at him. Then you "TICKLE" him and see how he responds.

"TICKLES" is the mnemonic for how to tell is a kid is truly sick. You will never be burned by using this. If you can assess a child with tickles and you find that they do not qualify for any of the mnemonic of tickles, they are not sick. This means they are not septic, they do not have a life-threatening problem going on in front of you, and you document this on the chart. T is tone. I is irritability. C is consolability. K is "kry." L is labor. E is environmental stimulation. S is skin.

T	**TONE**
I	**IRRITABILITY**
C	**CONSOLABILITY**
K	**KRY (CRY)**
L	**LABOR**
E	**ENVIRONMENTAL STIMULATION**
S	**SKIN**

When assessing a sick child, you want to look at the tone of the child. Is this child flailing their extremities around, pushing your hands away, or pushing your stethoscope away? This is a child with good tone and does not suggest a severely ill child (irritability to provoking examiner). A good example here is any time you look at a child's ears, they are not going to like that, or 9 out of 10 times, they will not be too happy with you. You have to hold their arms down, and they will fight you. This is a normal response. Another way to denote irritability is from a needle stick. If you are going to draw blood, you prick the kid, and they have a wimpy cry and do not respond much to the needle stick, that is a very ominous finding. C is for consolability by parents. This is when you are the bad medical provider, you just examined the ear, the child is crying, when you are done mom picks him up and he quiets down, and is happy and content in mom's arms. Again, that does not suggest a sick child. With regard to the kry, is it weak or strong? Is this someone who with a wimpy cry, or is this a loud, vigorous (annoy the whole emergency room) cry. If they have a loud and vigorous cry, they are not sick.

Labor is where we want to look at the breathing patterns.

Children represent sickness through their breathing. Are they breathing fast? Do they have retractions where you can see the ribs? Do they have nasal flaring and grunting? Grunting suggests auto "peep," and this will be discussed more in the respiratory chapter. As with the inspiratory to expiratory ratio, and again this will be discussed more in the respiratory chapter. E is environmental. How well are they responding to the environment? This is a child who will actually walk around the bed and walk around the parent while I am examining him or while I am just sizing them up for the look. Is this someone who is tracking me with their eyes. So, if I dangle keys out, is this a child who is going to turn his head and look at the keys versus someone who is just not stimulated by the environment at all? That is a much more ominous finding. A child who will look at me and watch me with his eyes, with a little bit of suspicion, is having a normal physiologic response that a child will have and this reaction does not denote a child who is truly sick.

With little babies, there is what is called the Moro response. As a little neonator infant, they will not necessarily be tracking you with their eyes, but if you take a finger and lightly graze either side of their cheek, this will stimulate a feeding response and will turn their head toward your finger to suckle, kind of like it was a nipple. The lack of that response denotes a child who will not eat, and this is concerning. Lastly is the skin. Is it moist? Is it cyanotic? Do they have a rash? Normal children will be moist and will not have cyanosis and no rash. With this mnemonic, I would also add in their feeding patterns. Children who are eating and drinking normally are not sick. Someone who has meningitis will not be eating and drinking normally.

Some notes about neonates, or children less than two months old. If you have a 2-month-old with a fever or a 6-week-old where you do a rectal temperature and get a reading of 102˚, this is an automatic septic work up. At the very least, they need I.V., chest x-ray, blood work, and urine from a catheterized specimen. Most likely, they will need a lumbar puncture as well. But, with these patients I will have a very low threshold to put antibiotics on board quickly.

There are academics in medicine that feel strongly that you should not put antibiotics on board until you have cultures done, meaning blood cultures, urine cultures and cerebral spinal fluid. I remember about 12 years ago in my training, I went on morning rounds, and a young physician was talking about child they had admitted the night before; how they had a really tough time getting a lumbar puncture done and therefore delayed antibiotics until the lumbar puncture was done. He, thinking he was a good doctor and a good resident, said that after a couple hours they finally got the lumbar puncture and then put antibiotics on board. He went on to describe the events of the following evening, and at the end of his presentation one of the physicians who was just getting off that morning, having worked the night shift, said "Hey, that child died." I remember the shock in the room. I remember walking away from that room and asking one of the senior residents why this happened. Why did it take so long to get antibiotics on board? He said he missed the forest from the trees. He was taught in medicine to give antibiotics when they are potentially life saving. So, from my perspective, when I see a child or someone in the emergency room whom I feel is septic and potentially has a life-threatening infection, I have a very low threshold to at the very least get a urine culture, blood culture and then put antibiotics on board right away, even before I call a specialist. It may make the diagnosis of this germ more difficult down the road, but in the process I may save their life. A buzzword here is Rocephin 50 mg per kg. Any child you think is life-threateningly sick, 50 mg per kg of Rocephin I.V. or I.M. is a potentially life-saving dose of antibiotic.

It is not uncommon to see a child in the emergency room where the presence of a life-threatening infection is not found, yet the diagnosis is uncertain. They get completely worked up to include cultures. They do not look too sick, meaning they are still irritable but the chest x-ray looks good, urine looks good, blood work looks good, and it is not uncommon to give a 50 mg per kg I.M. injection and have them follow up the next day to see how they doing, either in the office or back at the emergency room. At that time, if the cultures are not back, they will get a second injection of the 50 mg per kg Rocephin, just pending all those cultures. So, it is not uncommon to treat pediatric patients as out-patient using I.M. Rocephin.

From an antibiotic perspective, I want to talk about a case study. I want to talk about antibiotics and antibiotic selection, and if you think it is appropriate in this case. Imagine, the initial nurse triage notes included a date of 11/20/97, 9:40 a.m. with a temperature of 97.9° orally, pulse of 102, respirations of 18, and blood pressure of 150/94. The patient admits to being on cough drops. The triage information was, "I have a cold in my upper respiratory area." The patient complained of feeling short of breath. The nurse also documents cold symptoms x 5 days with increased temperature. The same nurse noted "wheezing in his lungs" and a pulse oximetry of 100% on room air. Also "alteration in comfort secondary to respiratory difficulties, MDP to evaluate and respiratory treatment." It was also noted, "Improvement from treatment. Discharge instructions given to patient, will comply." So imagine the medical note written as, "56-year-old white male complaining of upper respiratory infection symptoms x 4 days, no shortness of breath yet feels 'chest congestion.' No fevers or chills, no chest pain, pressure or palpitations. The patient stated that he walked 30 minutes on a treadmill yesterday. He feels that his symptoms have plateaued over the past two days. He said he spoke with his primary care physician who sent him to the emergency room secondary to meeting with him tomorrow." No dyspnea on exertion. Drinking well. Dyspnea is secondary to chest congestion. Wife also had the same symptoms yet resolved after three days. No medications, no allergies, no past medical history and a nonsmoker. Under objective, vital signs were stable other than a mild increase in blood pressure. His HEENT exam was within normal limits. Tympanic membranes bilaterally clear. Respiratory status included wheezing in upper and lower fields, no rales (clear to auscultation post-treatment). Going down further, his cardiovascular system showed regular rate and rhythm. Abdomen was soft and nontender. This gentleman was diagnosed with bronchitis and placed on Biaxin 500 mg twice per day for 10 days, and he was to follow up with his primary care physician.

So, the question is whether the antibiotic selection was correct. Would you have done anything different with this patient? Would you have done a chest x-ray or gotten blood work? This is an actual patient that I saw two months after graduating from PA school in 1997. The patient stands out in my mind because this patient actually died eight days later from a massive heart attack. This case went through the whole legal process of deposition and took years and years to finally conclude. It was suggested that I missed acute coronary syndrome presentation in a patient, and this could have proven to be a multi-million dollar lawsuit, which was ultimately dismissed with no findings of malpractice. The biggest reason that it was found in my favor because of documentation in my note.

We are using this case as an introduction to chest pain and chest symptoms and how to evaluate patients with pulmonary symptoms and to make sure we are not missing a life-threatening infection. With any patient who presents with chest symptoms, you have to assume it is a first tier, high-risk, can't miss life-threatening problem, such as I did with this patient. You have to assume it is cardiac and rule out cardiac by history or by diagnostic testing, and if you still cannot rule them out, you need to get someone smarter than you involved such as a cardiologist or get a consult.

Chapter 4

CHEST PAIN AND CARDIAC ENZYMES

When anyone comes in with chest symptoms, whether it is chest pain, pressure, shortness of breath, indigestion or cough, you have to ask, "Who is your PAPPA?" You need to look at them, point to them and say, "Who's your PAPPA?" PAPPA is a mnemonic for the high-risk, can't-miss cause of chest pain. If you miss it and they go home, they could die. So, these are the high-risk, can't-miss causes. Trust me when I say that you do not want to come to work and have someone say to you, "Hey, remember that patient you saw the other day" … because these conversations never end positively. It's rarely that they sent you a happy note. More commonly it is that the patient was admitted to another hospital with something bad, or came back with something bad.

PAPPA stands for high-risk, can't-miss causes of chest pain. The first two, PA, have to do with the heart. The next two, PP, have to do with the lungs. And the last A has to do with an aneurysm. P is pericarditis, A is acute coronary syndrome, P is pneumothorax, P is pulmonary embolism, and A is aneurysm.

P	**PERICARDITIS**
A	**ACUTE CORONARY SYNDROME**
P	**PNEUMOTHORAX**
P	**PULMONARY EMBOLISM**
A	**ANEURYSM**

Pericarditis almost always is viral. About 99% of the time it is viral, even though anything can inflame the pericardial sac, be it mechanical, traumatic or blood. It could be from uremia. So, multiple things can cause pericarditis, but 99 out of 100 times it is a virus. This only happens in young, healthy people. Patients classically complain of positional chest pain, meaning it hurts more when they lie down and feels much better when they sit upright. This has to do with the anatomy of the heart being kind of tugged on when lying flat and relieved when sitting up (gallbladder disease and gastroesophageal reflux disease also have symptoms that are worse with supine posture).

The diagnosis really hinges on the EKG, and the diffuse S-T segment elevations, which will be covered under the EKG portion of this book. Erythrocyte sedimentation rate is helpful under these circumstances. The work up is an echocardiogram to make sure they do not have a pericardial effusion. Beck's triad, which stands for muffled heart sounds, pulses paradoxes and jugular venous distention, is also a classic finding on board exams in someone with pericardial effusion. Understand that pulses paradoxes has to do with a drop in systolic blood pressure while a patient is taking in a deep breath. This is clinically of very low relevance. On board exams, if somebody has jugular venous distention, they have a problem with blood getting into the heart from one reason or another. The most common are congestive heart failure in that blood is not flowing in through the superior vena cava well, or pericardial tamponade because the heart is being squeezed, and blood is not going in or tension pneumothorax. So, if you see jugular venous distention you have to entertain one of those three diagnoses. The treatment for pericarditis is anti-inflammatory medication such as Motrin or Indocin and under severe circumstances, steroids.

Coronary artery disease (acute myocardial infarction or cardiac ischemia) is the number one killer of men in America. Coronary artery disease presents in patients in multiple ways. You can have someone come in who is so sick no one could miss the diagnosis. They are ashen gray, writhing around with chest pain, are sweaty and looking like they are on death's door. No one can miss that diagnosis. Someone else can come in and say they have indigestion. Those patients are so grossly atypical from a presentation of acute coronary syndrome, but you have to entertain this in anybody with chest symptoms. I would like to give you some pros on how to make sure you do not get burned and miss something tragic. 99% of the time the etiology of coronary artery disease is blood clot. Vasospasm of a coronary vessel can happen and is called Prinzmetal angina, though it is quite uncommon. So, 99.9% of the time, it is a blood clot.

History is the most important factor in the work up, treatment and evaluation of someone with cardiac ischemia. EKG is nice. Lab values are nice, but most hinges on history. You get the history of the events of the chest pain and a good assessment of risk factors. History. History. History. Any person who is reading this book right now, if they came in with chest pain and saw me in the emergency room, and they had a good story, they would be admitted at least for a 24-hour admission to have the chest pain worked up in greater detail. I have admitted countless number of patients to the hospital for an acute coronary syndrome work up even though their diagnostic tests were inconclusive or non-diagnostic.

Let's talk about some high-risk factors associated with acute coronary syndrome or cardiac ischemia. Exertional pain. If someone comes in saying they have chest symptoms when they exert themselves, it is angina until proven otherwise. It is classic that a gentleman can get chest pain when he shovels his driveway for the first time of the winter, or he mows the lawn and gets shortness of breath or chest pain. I had a patient I admitted to the hospital who came in complaining of indigestion and heartburn. I initially sent a student in to see this patient. He came out and said to put him on a proton-pump inhibitor and send him home. When I went in and got a full story, the patient said this indigestion was worse when he walked uphill. He noticed it over the past 2-3 days when he walked to work. He had to walk up a hill, which is when the indigestion seemed to hit him. So, in my mind, this presented as classic unstable angina. He was sent right away for cardiac catheterization where he had a 99% blockage of his left anterior descending artery, and I received this most amazing letter from his wife thanking me for saving her husband's life. This literally brought tears to my eyes. So, exertional chest pain is angina until proven otherwise.

Taking this a step further, exertional pain is ischemia. If someone comes in with severe calf pain while walking the mall, you have to assume that they have blockages in their peripheral vasculature so blood flow is not getting to their calf when they exert themselves. So, claudication or pain when they exert themselves suggests ischemia of the leg muscle. A very trick diagnosis is ischemic bowel. These are people who have blocked blood vessels to their bowel wall. They will present a lot of times with just diffuse abdominal pain that is out of proportion with the exam. Really bad mesenteric ischemia or mesenteric infarct will present writhing in pain yet when examining their belly, it is not too severe. People with mesenteric ischemia classically have abdominal pain about half hour to 90 minutes after eating because the food will get down to their intestines, and the blood flow tries to pick up to digest the food, but it is blocked. So, the bowel wall is not getting the blood supply it needs, and the patient will have terrible pain. I would suggest to you folks that some of the worst pain I have seen, as a provider, has to do with ischemia to the heart, the belly, or the leg and from kidney stones or gallstones. These are some of the worst pains I have seen in my career. I guess generally you could say, if something is being blocked and not allowing normal physiology to occur the body freaks out at that and knows it is going to die if you don't fix it.

In talking about high-risk factors from an historic perspective about acute coronary syndrome, you have to look at the character of the pain. Typically the pain is more of a pressure, an ache, a dullness. People say it feels like someone pushing on their chest. This has to do with the visceral nerves and how they innervate the spine. If they innervate at multiple different levels, they feel a vague pressure. When people have muscle pain or pulmonary pain, it innervates the spine at one specific nerve fiber and the patient feels the pain more as sharp or pinpoint.

Diaphoresis is also important with pain. If someone has pain and breaks out in a sweat, always consider this very severe. I am telling you this from my years working as a house officer. The nurses may call saying, "Mrs. Smith has belly pain and broke out into a sweat." or, "Mr. Smith had chest pain and got sweaty". This is always something severe. I can say this is when they had a myocardial infarction, pulmonary embolism, aneurysm rupture, or a peptic ulcer that has popped. So, if you have someone who comes in with severe symptoms or significant symptoms and they broke out into a sweat, I can say that clinically I have found that a very ominous finding.

Most recently I had someone come in with a syncopal episode. It was an elderly lady who basically was talking to her kids and suddenly fell over right into her cereal. She was unresponsive for a number of minutes until the EMS got there. They found her grossly sweaty and pale. When they brought her in, however, she was completely normal. By the time she got to us, she looked good and felt well. She did not have chest pain but did pass out and was grossly sweaty. In my mind, I was confident that this was either an arrhythmia or an intracranial hemorrhage. When in the emergency room, all of a sudden she went unresponsive again and went from a sinus rhythm to a complete heart block to asystole. This lasted about 20-30 seconds, then her intrinsic rhythm kicked back in, and she came back alive. This happened twice. So, once again, I tell you to take diaphoresis and chest or abdominal pain. very seriously

Shortness of breath with pain is common with acute coronary syndrome as is nausea and vomiting. Nausea and vomiting is typically seen more with inferior wall issues where on the lower portion of the heart that has a tendency to irritate the diaphragm and the vagus nerve more than other areas of the heart. They typically get sick to their stomach or even throw up. The time frame interval for acute coronary syndrome has to do with hours, not minutes. It is not someone who says they had pain that came and went in 30 seconds. That is very atypical in someone with acute coronary syndrome.

If you think of the pathophysiology of ischemia, it has to do with a blocked blood vessel that has a thrombus that gets progressively worse. It is not an embolism and not a clot that floats and dams everything up all at once, not like a pulmonary embolism. This is a clot that grows and grows. (Everybody has some degree of atherosclerosis over the age of 30; it is not likely for anyone to have 100% patent coronary artery.) But let's just say we have a completely patent coronary artery and a blood clot starts, let's say for the sake of this book that with an 80% blockage, you will have chest pain. So, the blood clot starts at 50%, maybe you just feel vague, just don't feel well and a bit more short of breath. All of a sudden you hit 80% and start getting a chest pressure. As that progresses to 90%, you get severe pressure. Then, at 100% you get your myocardial infarction. So, understand that the chest pain from acute coronary syndrome normally goes on for hours, not minutes or seconds. Radiation of pain north to northeast should be an ominous finding, whether it is pain going into the shoulder, the neck, or the left arm. I did have a patient who was a relatively young guy at 62. He came in with cough and some chest symptoms that made his chest hurt a bit more when he took deep breaths. He was a rheumatoid arthritis patient, saying that his rheumatoid arthritis was a little worse than normal and his teeth hurt. I asked what he meant by his teeth hurt, and he said, "My teeth ache." I asked whether he ever had dental problems before, to which he answered, "no." It was from that history of weird chest symptoms and dental pain that I evaluated him for a cardiac etiology. His cardiac enzymes indeed came back positive. So, without any question, this patient had a myocardial infarction. The only thing that saved me was thinking that the pain in his teeth was a radiation of pain north.

Some low risk factors for cardiac ischemia have to do with positional or pleuritic chest pain, positional meaning it hurts more when moving, pleuritic meaning it hurts more when breathing. Either it is purely pleuritic meaning that it only hurts when breathing or partially pleuritic meaning it hurts more when breathing. Picture this; if someone has a tack on the inner wall of their lung, and the only time that tack pokes the lung is when taking a deep breath, they will say it only hurts when breathing, opposed to someone who has broken ribs which hurts all the time but more when breathing. So, is it purely pleuritic or partially pleuritic. Sharp stabbing pain, as described earlier, has to do with one nerve innervating the spine at one spot. Again, the timing of the pain is important. Is it minutes to seconds- which is less likely to be cardiac? Is it reproducible with palpation? I would use this as a very crude guide. There are clear cases documented in people who say it hurts when pushing, if pushing right here, it hurts more. They indeed have a cardiac etiology of their chest pain, and I can say that I have clinically seen that, where you can push on their chest and it hurts more. It moves them more into a low-risk classification in your mind yet does not mean absolute that it is no. Gastrointestinal symptoms, again, do not mean that it is not cardiac but puts it in a lower risk pool.

As I talked about the patient before who had gastrointestinal symptoms with exertion, and I know from reviewing medical-legal literature, it is a classic law suit if someone has indigestion, present to the emergency department, got a gastrointestinal cocktail and felt better, and they were sent home, subsequently dying. This is classic. It is an important point to say that therapeutic challenge is never diagnostic which means if you give someone a gastrointestinal cocktail and they feel better, it does not mean it is their stomach, just as if you give someone nitroglycerin and their chest pain feels better, it does not mean it is their heart. Now, this is not just important from a medical-legal perspective, it is important for you as a clinician. The placebo effect means that the body will act a certain way when the patient believes something is going to help them. It is classic. If you start someone on a new medication, let's say for hair growth, 1/3 of all patients who take the medication are going to grow hair even if it is a placebo just based on the normal physiologic placebo response. So, once again, if you give someone a gastrointestinal cocktail and they feel better, does that mean it is gastrointestinal? No, it does not mean it is gastrointestinal. Is it helpful? Of course it is helpful. It would not show you are using all of your resources if you did not weigh that into your considerations, but is it possible for people with ischemic chest pain to feel better after the gastrointestinal cocktail? Absolutely it is. So, from a medical-legal perspective and as a clinician, you have to remember this term that therapeutic challenge is never diagnostic.

Once again, history is the most important factor in working up a patient. Not just with the historical features of the chest pain as we described above. We have to talk about cardiac risk factors, and I have never been one to be able to remember lists so I have to come up with mnemonics for everything. So, for cardiac risk factors, I say that is a **SAD** case of **CHF**.

S	**SMOKING**
A	**AGE**
D	**DIABETES**
C	**CHOLESTEROL**
H	**HYPERTENSION**
F	**FAMILY HISTORY**

S is smoking. A is age. D is diabetes. C is cholesterol. H is hypertension. F is family history. Remember some important points about the cardiac risk factors. Always encourage patients to stop smoking no matter why they are in the emergency room or why they are seeing you at your family practice. I do think a lot of times it is moot, and it is tough to get people to change their behavior, but as a provider I want what's best for my patients. Just because I don't think they will do it does not mean that I am going to change my approach. A healthy patient is a patient who does not smoke. I want all my patients to be healthy so I am going to encourage every patient to not smoke. Age typically means greater than 55 for a male and greater than 65 for a female.

D is diabetes. It is now thought that if you have diabetes, you have coronary artery disease. We used to consider it the worst risk factor someone could have for coronary artery disease, now it is more thought that if you have a 50-year-old male with diabetes and they come in with chest pain, you automatically have to put them in a very high risk pool for having unstable angina. If they have diabetes and chest pain, they automatically go to a very high-risk pool. Cholesterol, high cholesterol and poorly controlled cholesterol, hypertension, family history which is really important (looking for first degree relatives who had coronary artery disease at a young age) in looking for genetic predisposition. There are some other less tangible risk factors for heart disease such as obesity. When you ask that question, you have to determine who is obese, what classifies someone who is obese. I would like to suggest that obese people have a higher incidence of high blood pressure, high cholesterol and diabetes and go more by those objective findings. We also say a Type A personality has a high risk of coronary artery disease. Again, this is very difficult to objectively measure. Sedentary lifestyle is also difficult to measure. I would recommend going by SAD CHF and documenting them on the chart.

You need to weigh into all of your decision making the fact that atypical presentations occur. Most commonly in the literature, this occurs in females, elderly and diabetics. Younger women, in their 30s, who come in with weird chest symptoms. Elderly women fall into a classification for following atypically because of being elderly, so that is a second class of patients, but not just because they are female. So, it is normally younger females, the elderly and diabetics. Know that diabetic nerve innervations of the heart and intestines are different. Their nerves have gotten fried over the years, and they just do not respond normally. So if a diabetic comes in and says they just don't feel well, you have to entertain that this could be cardiac ischemia and work up appropriately (diabetics can also have non-diagnostic abdominal exams as we discussed in the first chapter).

Here are some examples of atypical presentations. I had a gentleman come in who was in his 40s. He presented by ambulance with a chief complaint of weakness. When the patient came in, he was sitting on a stretcher looking happy as a clam, smiling, kind of waving to me. I was thinking that this guy looks way too good to come in here by ambulance. He looks too happy and is enjoying this too much. When I talked to the paramedics, they said he has been weak and has been unable to get off the couch for the past three days. Again, in my mind I was thinking that this guy just didn't want to go to work or was being lazy and looked way too good to have that degree of symptoms and come in by ambulance. When I went in to see the patient he told me he was weak and could not get off the couch. I asked, "You haven't been able to get off the couch for three days?" He said, "yes." I thought I would trick him and asked how he was going to the bathroom. He responded by saying he had to pee in a bottle. So, at this point he got my attention.

I asked him what he meant by being weak. He said that every

time he took a step he got short of breath. Now, he really has my attention. So, we basically started a cardiac work up. A cardiac work up demands an EKG be performed promptly. When the EKG was put in front of me, it looked like this guy had a relatively acute inferior wall myocardial infarction with S-T segment elevations and Q-wave formations. So, now I am wondering why this guy would have symptoms of being weak and no other symptoms of chest pain. I gave the patient a really good questionnaire about gastrointestinal symptoms or neck pain or belly pain, something that would say he had this infarction. He said, "Nope, nothing." With that, I wondered what would make this guy present as an atypical chest pain. I had the nurse check his fingerstick, and his blood sugar was 300. He told us that he had not seen a doctor in 10 years. So, this was a classic silent myocardial infarction in a diabetic.

Most recently I had a woman come in to the emergency room with a hypoglycemic episode. As we worked her up, all of her findings appeared nonspecific, and we admitted her to watch this hypoglycemic episode. An attending physician nudged me to check an EKG and some cardiac enzymes and, to my embarrassment, her cardiac enzymes came back positive. Therefore, this patient had a hypoglycemic episode because of a myocardial infarction.

The most satisfying cardiac arrest I worked was a 36-year-old female who came in. We had a really busy emergency room, and she presented by ambulance with an episode of having had a seizure. When she arrived at the emergency room, we put her in the back just because we were so busy with some pretty severely ill patients. When I went to see her, she had another seizure while she was on the stretcher. The paramedics were still there, so I asked whether she had a seizure history, and they responded with a no. By the time she came out of the seizure, which lasted 5-10 seconds, she was not breathing and was not responding like a typical postictal patient.

Quickly we whipped her into one of our cardiac rooms, and she was in ventricular tachycardia. The code ended up lasting 90 minutes between multiple shocks and multiple different medications, until finally we got a viable blood pressure back and we stabilized her. A 12-lead EKG demonstrated that she was indeed having an acute anterior wall infarction. She got thrombolytics and was flown out of our small rural emergency department, shocked multiple times in the helicopter, and was cardiac catheterized and stented. I ended up seeing her months later to be admitted for pancreatitis. When we reviewed the chart and literature on her history, she had been having waxing and waning chest symptoms over the prior couple of months and was seen in her physician's office multiple times and also seen in the emergency room. So, this is a classic example of a young female with chest pain that was cardiac in nature.

Any young patient with chest pain (I have seen this more with guys) has a very low threshold until you do a toxicology screen looking for a drugs such as cocaine or crack. Most patients will not admit to this, but will come in with chest symptoms. So, now you have a 25-year-old male who comes in with chest pain. You do a toxicology screen and find out they are indeed positive for cocaine. You have to take them very seriously and need to be admitted for further evaluation. You don't just say to stop the cocaine and it will go away. No, they need to be admitted and taken very seriously because they have a high incidence of sudden death.

A normal EKG means nothing. If you have an ominous or an ischemic appearing EKG, the patient is admitted, and it is an easy case. A normal EKG means nothing, so have a low threshold to do, at the very least, two EKGs on the patient and make sure there are no changes. It still comes down to the story. EKGs are indeed quite helpful if you see dynamic changes. For example, if you see S-T segment changes or T-wave inversions that have changed over a period of time.

I had a young man who came in to see us in the emergency room with chest pain that had very atypical features. It hurt more when he bent over, hurt more when he took deep breaths. But, he was a smoker and he had us concerned enough that we worked him up in the emergency room. All of his enzymes were negative, and his EKG x2 were normal. So, I talked to his physician, had him set up to have a stress test done in two days and placed him on the appropriate medications. He actually came back to the emergency room approximately 1½ days later with a massive anterior wall myocardial infarction. He had to have cardiac catheterization and had a left ventricle that was destroyed by the infarction. He then went on to have a heart transplant. I reviewed the case, and all my colleagues went back and reviewed the case. It never made its way into the legal system, but was gone over with a fine-tooth comb.

Any time that something goes bad in medicine, you really need to be your own worst critic. You need to look at it and ask yourself what you could have done better or differently. How can I take better care of patients the next time? As an educator, I looked at this case and asked, "What can I learn from this case and teach students so they never make this same mistake or this never happens again?" I went to one of my colleagues (Michael Woltz) who reviewed the case in detail. Michael is a true, shoot-from-the-hip kind of guy and has a way of saying that you really dropped the ball. He gives feedback that is appropriate. He basically reviewed the chart in detail, and I asked what I could learn or take away from this. His advice was that sometimes you can do everything right and still bad things happen. Obviously, I found this quite reassuring.

Cardiac enzymes and Troponin (what does Willie Sutton say? Willie Sutton says Troponin is where the money is). Troponin is the best and most sensitive of all the cardiac markers. There are two different isoforms, the I-isoform and the T-isoform. Both have mild differences between them and some labs use different isoforms. They both do the same thing. If they have cardiac injury, the troponin will be high. Therefore, if someone has a positive troponin, they indeed have had a myocardial infarction to some degree.

The troponin normally rises about 30 to 90 minutes after injury and stays up for approximately 10-14 days. Normal value is approximately less than 1.5, yet different labs have different reference ranges. Now, the elevation of troponin is clinically significant to the degree of damage. So, a troponin of 7 or 8 is less ominous than a troponin of 70 or 80. Now, typically when somebody is admitted to the hospital and they have a positive troponin in the emergency department, the troponins are still monitored to see where they peak and where they come down. So, if a troponin in the emergency room is 5, they are admitted and six hours later the troponin is 12, the troponin six hours after that is back to 6, they would say the troponin maximum was 12. If the third value keeps climbing, that suggests more significant myocardial damage than first thought. Be aware that micro damage of the heart such as seen in congestive heart failure or unstable angina will mildly bump the troponin up.

An example of this would be a 49-year-old white female who presents with an episode of chest pain while mowing the lawn. She comes in to the emergency room, and the first troponin is negative. She is admitted to the hospital and a second troponin is positive to 2.0. Then the third troponin at 12 hours is negative again, so less than 1.5. This patient would be diagnosed with a positive AMI and would go on to get cardiac evaluation and most likely a cardiac catheterization. A troponin maximum of 2.0 shows micro damage and clinically is not very impressive. Once, again a troponin of 30 is very significant for acute myocardial infarction. I personally have seen troponins as high as 180 which, the higher the troponin, the higher the mortality.

Another cardiac marker is creatinine kinase (creatinine

phosphokinase or CPK). This is an enzyme that is found in all muscle tissue, be it skeletal or cardiac. There are a couple isoenzymes that are available that may help us clinically. There is the isoenzyme MM, which is found in muscle tissue, and the isoenzyme of MB, which is referred to as the CKMB. CKMB is specific to cardiac damage. This test was the primary test for acute coronary syndrome and myocardial infarction until about the late 80s, when the troponin came into use. The CK is really used for a secondary diagnostic test for acute coronary syndrome. How this test is used is a bit trickier and not as clear-cut as the troponin. There is a triad that needs to be in place in order to have the patient ruled in positive for an acute myocardial infarction using CPK. One is that the total CK has to be elevated. Second is the MB portion, the MB isoenzyme, needs to be elevated and the ratio being between the two needs to be greater than 5. Therefore, if we had a patient who came in with a total CK of 400 and an MB fraction of 40, both are elevated, and the ratio between the two is 10. So, 40 goes into 400 ten times and therefore you have a positive acute myocardial infarction as ruled in by CPKs.

CPK is also a test used to look for skeletal muscle damage known as rhabdomyolysis. This is typically seen with prolonged immobilization. It can also be seen with electric shock or crush injuries. Basically, it denotes severe death of skeletal muscles in a rapid period of time. Clinically, this is most commonly seen in elderly folks who fall on the floor and are not found for 6-12 hours. Normally, if someone sleeps on the floor they have a normal physiologic response, when their muscles start becoming ischemic, they shift position during sleep to compensate for that muscle being ischemic. If someone is debilitated, sick or for some reason do not have those protective mechanisms, the muscles will indeed die, necrose and secrete CPK.

In the case of Electric shock, (where an impulse goes through the body like a bullet) there is an entrance wound and an exit wound. I have seen shock victims- one person in particular who had electric shock from metal girder that touched an overhead wire while it was being moved by a crane. The electric shock went through his hand and when he came in, we actually smelled burning flesh. We took off his shoe and saw the scorch mark out his heel. So basically, the electricity went through his hand, through his body, and came out his heel. The problem is that when electricity zips through the body, it kills cells left and right, so there is significant rhabdomyolysis from this injury. Treatment is aggressive I.V. fluids, but we really need to be aware that the high protein load will dam up the kidneys and put them into renal failure. So, the treatment is very aggressive I.V. fluids and monitoring their ins and outs quite closely.

There is some degree of a therapeutic gray zone about using sodium bicarbonate. I have talked with internists about this. This can vary from a patient who has a medically induced rhabdomyolysis (such as someone with prolonged immobilization on the floor like grandma who fell and fractured her hip) versus someone who has an acute crush injury in an acute trauma setting. So, grandma who laid on the floor for 24 hours has rhabdomyolysis that developed over 24 hours, where the acute crush injury would have this relatively acute. I did talk to internists and trauma surgeons about this. Trauma surgeons are a little quicker to pull the trigger in using sodium bicarbonate and the I.V. fluids. The internist is a little less aggressive with that. As a midlevel, I would defer judgment and go with what the specialists tell me to do.

The last cardiac marker I will make you aware of is myoglobin. It is very sensitive yet not very specific. When I say this, I mean if someone has a myocardial infarction at time 0, there is muscle damage. The heart has been damaged. Myoglobin will be the first cardiac enzyme to elevate. The problem with this is that if someone has a high myoglobin, it could be high in any muscle in the body. I have seen children come in after football practice with very high myoglobins because they kept getting tackled and their muscles were damaged. So myoglobin is very sensitive, it is just not very specific. If someone comes in, by ambulance, with a severe episode of chest pain, (with bloods drawn at bedside by the paramedics) and the troponin is normal, and the myoglobin is maybe 2-3 times normal, that could suggest an acute myocardial infarction, just that the troponin has not had time to catch up with it. Once again, the myoglobin will rise first. The CPK will rise second and the troponin third. When we talk about this, there is a bit of difference in time as to how fast they go up. I can say clinically that I have seen this way too many times, myoglobins first, CPKs second and troponins third. Normally, we are talking 30-45 minute interval between the two. So, if someone comes in with an acute episode of chest pain and we drew their labs within 30 minutes, let's say the myoglobin, which is very nonspecific, is mildly elevated but CPK and troponin are negative, we will sit on them in the emergency room and recheck the labs in two hours. If the CPK and the troponin are still normal, you can have a high degree of confidence that this was not a myocardial infarction.

One time, in teaching laboratory medicine at a physician assistant school, I had a PA bowl where I asked the class to submit five questions on 3x5 cards, on one side of the sheet there was the question, and on the other side there was the answer. I had one interesting student ask the question, "If you were a cardiac enzyme, which would your girlfriend rather you be?" (It was my fault that I did not pre-screen these questions to avoid a degree of embarrassment.) The answer turned out to be, "It depends because a myoglobin is more sensitive yet a troponin stays up longer." Entertaining and embarassing, yet did teach a significant point that is not soon forgotten by students. Myoglobin is very nonspecific and is up and down relatively quickly. It spikes and then leaves the system.

Troponin will stay positive for about a week. So, someone who is admitted to the hospital with an acute myocardial infarction, they have a cardiac catheterization, discharged on day 3 and come back on day 7, you run labs and they have a positive troponin, you have to ask whether this is a new myocardial infarction or is the troponin just raised from the last admission.

The bottom line is that troponin is the best test for acute myocardial infarction and cardiac ischemia. One negative test is not enough. We need at least two diagnostic tests, with a couple of hours between each, to prove there was no myocardial infarction. Normally, if we admit someone for acute chest pain, we will run three, at the very least, over a 6-8 hour interval.

In discussing cardiac disease, this is an appropriate time to talk about congestive heart failure. The cardiac lab test to assess left ventricular function is called a beta natriuretic, also known as BNP. This is a relatively new test that looks at ventricular stretch. The higher the BNP, the worse the congestive heart failure. A normal value is approximately 180. This test is helpful in assessing someone's shortness of breath, especially if you have a patient with combination diagnoses of chronic obstructive pulmonary disease and congestive heart failure, and they come in short of breath. Your concern is whether this is primarily a congestive heart failure issue or more of a chronic obstructive pulmonary disease issue, which would require a very different treatment. In discussing congestive heart failure, the primary cause of congestive heart failure is ischemic heart disease, where someone could have blocked blood vessels to the heart, and when those are corrected with angioplasty or coronary artery bypass graft. The second most common cause is hypertensive cardiac disease that puts a patient into failure.

From an academic perspective, the paradigm with congestive heart failure used to be that of mechanical issue with the heart. Now, when we look at congestive heart failure, we evaluate preload, load and after-load. Preload has to do with the water coming into a bucket. Load has to do with the pump taking the water out of the bucket. After-load has to do with the hose with which you are pumping the water out of the bucket. We used to think in terms very mechanically of decreasing preload with diuretics, making the pump work better with positive ionotrobes, such as digoxin. Then we would decrease after-load by making the hose larger that is pumping out the bucket- with ace inhibitors or morphine.

Rather than thinking of congestive heart failure as a mechanical issue, we are now treating it more as a neurohormonal issue, where if we can decrease the hormonal influence on the heart, we can have patients live longer. The mainstays in therapy are beta-blockers and ace inhibitors. If you have a patient with congestive heart failure and they are not on a beta-blocker or ace inhibitor, you are deviating from a standard of care. The evidence is strong that patients on ace inhibitors and beta-blockers live longer lives.

From an emergency perspective, when it comes to a patient coming into the emergency room with congestive heart failure, we as clinicians need to make the appropriate diagnosis where the beta natriuretic peptide and a chest x-ray is helpful. Treatment is what I would like to spend a little time talking about. The mnemonic I used to use for treating congestive heart failure was the letters of the alphabet, **LMNOP**.

L	**LASIX**
M	**MORPHINE**
N	**NITRATES**
O	**OXYGEN**
P	**PEE**

Congestive heart failure: L is Lasix. M is morphine. N is nitrates. O is oxygen. P stands for pee- what they do after receiving Lasix. Let's say someone comes into the emergency room and they are moderately ill. They have kind of a guppy breathing, have broken sentences, are sweaty, and definitely anxious, but they are alert and oriented x3. In these patients, I would typically have the nurse get an I.V. line in and give high-flow oxygen. While I am waiting for the nurse to get good I.V. access, I would put nitro paste on them. At that point, once I.V. access is in place, we would initiate diuretic therapy and nitroglycerin I.V. as well as different aliquots of morphine.

In discussing these three treatment modalities, there is one that stands out far and above the other two. Nitroglycerin is your money here. It is the medication that is going to make your patients feel best the fastest. And, you need to hit them high with a nitro-drip. Typically nitroglycerin drip from acute coronary perspectives, we start at 5-10 mCg per minute. Congestive heart failure patients need much more than that. You need to start at 40, 50 or 60. Now, this will typically make the nursing staff nervous but understand still that if for some reason you start to bottom out the pressure, nitroglycerin I.V. has a very short half-life and you can turn it off. On a comparative note, if a patient took three sublingual nitroglycerin per 5 minutes, a nitroglycerin tablet is 0.4 mg or 400 mCg, so if you have them take three of those tablets over 10 minutes because you would have them taking nitroglycerin at x0, x5 minutes and x10 minutes, that is 1200 mCg in approximately 10 minutes. Now, you get about 75-80% absorption with nitroglycerin, so if you are absorbing 75% of one tablet, for every tablet of 400 mCg, a patient is absorbing approximately 300 mCg. After they take three tablets, they are ingesting approximately 900 mCg of nitroglycerin. If we start a patient at 10 mCg a minute of nitro I.V., it equates to 600 mCg per hour. If the patient took three, SL-Nitro at home and came in, they are already going to be reaching a state of about 900 mCg an hour. If we start them at 10 mCg per hour, that is 600 mCg per hour and that is already lower than what they took at home. So, do not hesitate to start higher with nitroglycerine.

When someone is in congestive heart failure, they get very low blood flow (approximately 20%) to the kidneys. Typically as a clinician, I would double their daily dose of Lasix, so if they are on 40 daily, I would give 80. Now remember that only about 20% of blood flow is going through their kidneys, so when you hit them with this heavier dose of Lasix, that Lasix is going to stay in circulation, just not just make its way to the kidney where it needs to work. Therefore, what happens is that these patients will start feeling better when you vasodilate them with the nitrates. After you vasodilate them, they start feeling better, and it is at that time that there will be full flow to the kidneys, and the Lasix will hit the kidneys and make these patients actually dehydrated.

Studies have shown that when patients present with congestive heart failure, 40-50 of them are dehydrated anyway. This goes against what I initially thought as a young provider. It was my understanding that any patient who is in congestive heart failure has fluid-overload. As I became more involved with critical care medicine, I have realized that is just not the case. When someone comes in in congestive heart failure, it is a redistribution issue more times than it is a fluid overload issue. An example of this would be someone who comes in with an acute myocardial infarction that puts them into pulmonary edema. These patients are happily going along with their day, and bam, they have a massive heart attack and are filled up with fluid. They are not hypervolemic they are uvolemic. So, again, if you pound them with diuretics, you are going to make them worse a day out because they are going to become hypotensive and need to replace fluid I.V. So with that said, I am not suggesting that we do not use diuretics in the treatment of acute congestive heart failure. I would suggest you hit them very hard with vasodilators such as nitrates, and once they start feeling better, hit them with smaller doses of Lasix such as 10-20 I.V.

Now, let's discuss morphine and using morphine with

congestive heart failure. Morphine was thought to be an anxiolytic and was used to decrease preload to a small degree, thus making patients a bit calmer and helping blood flow. More recent data shows that this is not as effective as once thought. I most recently heard a speaker stating that when you look at the data on morphine and congestive heart failure, it is "almost malpractice" to use it because there are no studies showing benefit. There are, however, a lot of studies showing that it does harm. Even though we still use it, the date looking at morphine really comes from the 70s, and peripheral veins being measured, not central circulation. It is from this most recent information that as a clinician I will never use morphine in congestive heart failure patients again, unless they are having an ischemic event as well and having chest pain, and then I would only use it as an analgesic. Morphine is an analgesic, not a hypnotic. It does not sedate people, even though at higher doses the side effect is sedation. Also, morphine can create quite an allergic response. I feel that morphine has a very low role in this day and age in treatment of acute congestive heart failure.

Digoxin is a medication used in two areas, congestive heart failure and atrial fibrillation. Digoxin is a positive inotropin and negative chromotrope, and this will be discussed more under the pharmacology chapter of this book.

Continuing on with our mnemonic of **PAPPA**, remember that **PAPPA** is a mnemonic for patients who come in with chest pain where the first two, PA, have to do with the heart, pericarditis and acute coronary syndrome. PP stands for the lungs, where P is pneumothorax and P is pulmonary embolism. Pneumothorax or traumatic pneumothorax quintessentially happens in tall, skinny males. They present with sudden, acute shortness of breath, often combined with chest pain. The risk is that this progresses to a tension pneumothorax, which is a life-threatening pulmonary problem. So always ask yourself,

"Who's your PAPPA?"

P	PERICARDITIS
A	ACUTE CORONARY SYNDROME
P	PNEUMOTHORAX
P	PULMONARY EMBOLISM
A	ANEURYSM

Pneumothorax is not uncommon in traumas such as car accidents, gunshot wounds and stab wounds, as well as falls. If a patient comes in with significant right- sided chest injury and you can feel crepitus and subcutaneous air on the right side of the chest, you do not need a chest x-ray to determine whether these people need a chest tube. You can go ahead and put it in because if they have chest trauma with subcutaneous air, you must transport them with a chest tube, because the life-threatening complication is indeed a tension pneumothorax. You can take that risk off the table just by prophylactically placing the tube. The best way to diagnose pneumothoraces is with a chest x-ray, and this can be ordered as an inspiratory/expiratory view.

As a student in PA school, I did have a 16-year-old male, a tall, skinny, marathon runner who came in with a spontaneous pneumothorax. I was a young, ambitious PA student really hoping to be able to put this chest tube in. He came in with a small, approximately 10% pneumothorax. He was observed overnight, and the plan was that if the pneumothorax resolved itself, he would go home the next day. If it got worse, he would need a chest tube. Being the young, ambitious person I was, I slept at the hospital that night so I could wake up in the morning and check the films. When I looked at the film it sure looked like the pneumothorax got better, so I went to the patient and family, who I became close with, and said it looked as though he should be able to go home. I then realized that the film I had looked at was the inspiratory film, not the expiratory film.

When we take a deep breath in, that expands the chest cavity but will also expand the lung. It is kind of like thinking of a balloon in a brown paper bag. The balloon is the lung itself, and the brown paper bag is the outer part of the lung or the parietal pleura of the sac hat the lung expands into. When someone takes a deep breath in, that is like blowing air into the balloon, and that balloon will expand out, filling the brown paper bag. The expiratory view means that the balloon will shrink up as much as it can, and if there is air between the balloon and the bag, that would suggest a pneumothorax. Now, when I looked at the inspiratory film with this young man taking a deep breath in, it sure looked like the pneumothorax resolved itself. However, when looking at the expiratory film, it was very clear that the pneumothorax indeed had gotten worse. When the doctor came in and looked at the film, it was clear that the pneumothorax had gotten worse. So, I actually had to go back and tell them that I had screwed up and that the pneumothorax was worse. He could not go home that day and actually needed a chest tube. They understood; but I sure learned the importance of inspiratory and expiratory radiographs.

Pulmonary embolism is the grim reaper of chest symptoms. "Where is the most common and consistent location to diagnose pulmonary embolism?" Is it in the family practice office? Is it in the emergency department? Is it in the radiology suite? Is in the pulmonologist's office? The answer is in the morgue and at autopsy. Pulmonary embolism is a deadly disease that is under-diagnosed, and when it is under-diagnosed, people die. It is a bad diagnosis. It is, once again, the grim reaper of chest symptoms. I gave this lecture in the past, and a student who worked in a morgue, came to me after class and said, "John, I was surprised at how many patients drop dead unexpectedly from pulmonary embolism." So, she saw that first-hand in the medical examiner's office.

Part of the reason that pulmonary embolism is such a vague

diagnosis or such a difficult diagnosis is because of the wide range of complaints patients can have when they present and the variety of problems it can create. It could be pleuritic chest pain or shortness of breath. It could be syncope. When someone comes in with shortness of breath, there are literally scores of things that it could be, including pneumonia, asthma, or infections like bronchitis. When we look at a patient like this, you don't ever want to make a **HORID** mistake and miss something.

H	**HEART**
O	**OBSTRUCTION**
R	**REACTIVE**
I	**INFECTION**
D	**DEATH (from Pulmonary embolism)**

H is heart. O is obstruction. Right is reactive. I is infection. D is death from a pulmonary embolism. This will be explained more under the radiology chapter. I would suggest that any patient who comes in with chest symptoms, whether it is shortness of breath, indigestion or chest pain, you have to rule out PAPPA and pulmonary embolism has to fall into that line of thought, use the HORID mnemonic This is as clear as someone with bronchitis. If someone comes in with bronchitis, coughing up white gooky stuff, the chances are 199/200 that it is a viral or maybe even bacterial bronchitis, which will respond to Proventil and maybe antibiotics. 1 out of 200, 1 out of 300. 1 out of 500 will be something bad such as an acute myocardial infarction or pulmonary embolism. They will present very atypically.

The key to diagnosis is risk factors. Now, the risk factors are best denoted as Virchow's triad. Virchow's triad has to do with hypercoagulability, damage to a blood vessel and stasis. Hypercoagulable states have to do with patients who are predisposed to foreign blood clots, such as patients with cancer or a history of cancer, a history of blood clots in themself or someone in the family, or someone with a high estrogen state such as pregnancy or on birth control pills. Damage to a blood vessel or near a blood vessel could be due to trauma such as a broken leg, knee surgery or an intravascular procedure of the lower extremity. What happens is when the vessel near this injury is irritated it has a tendency to form a blood clot. Stasis has to do with someone who is on bedrest or prolonged immobilization such as a long plane ride, someone who is debilitated in a hospital bed for a number of days and someone with a stroke.

When I am sizing someone up for pulmonary embolism risk factors, I will say to them, "Do you have a history of cancer? Have you or anybody in your family ever had a blood clot? Are you pregnant or have you been pregnant any time within the last couple of months? Have you been on any long trips recently such as on the plane or train, where you have been in a sedentary position for a while? Have you had any broken bones or surgery below your waist within the last couple of months? If the patient answers "no" to all of them, you can safely document on your chart, no Virchow's triad. It has been proven that patients can have pulmonary embolism without a documented risk factor. I have done case reviews multiple times in the past and had a part-time business doing medical-legal review. From a medical-legal perspective, if you document on the chart "no Virchow's triad" that tells a lawyer that you looked for it. You looked to see if this person might have pulmonary embolism. As we discussed earlier, pulmonary embolism is the grim reaper of chest symptoms, and people can just drop dead from it. If a person came in with asthma last week drops dead suddenly from pulmonary embolism, you should immediately assume legal action. However, when you document on the chart, long history of asthma and no Virchow's triad, you are telling people that you thought about that, asked about it and thought working them up for pulmonary embolism was not necessary. I highly recommend that with any patient who presents with chest symptoms, you MUST document cardiac risk factors, MUST document Virchow's triad and MUST document a leg exam.

Remember that deep venous thrombosis can let go and go to the lung. Most of the time, the leg is the origin of a blood clot. So, in evaluation fo pulmonary embolism, the two key components are documenting risk factors and documenting symmetrical legs, or no edema in one leg. Remember that with the leg exam, Homans sign suggests dorsiflexing the foot and pain in the calf suggests deep venous thrombosis. Understand that this is a relatively silly test. It has very low sensitivity or specificity but is a buzzword. If you look at textbooks, they talk about Homans sign being indicative of pulmonary embolism. Clinically, if you called me into the emergency room and said you had a patient with positive Homans sign and were sending them in for DVT work up, I would think you were probably well read but probably pretty new to medicine because it carries very little clinical weight. But, if you document on your chart no Homans sign, and I reviewed that chart, I would know that you specifically evaluated the leg for DVT. So, once again, if someone comes in with pulmonary symptoms that look like asthma or bronchitis, I cannot stress enough to document cardiac risk factors: document no Virchow's triad, document no edema in the legs and no Homans sign. That will provide a very legally defensible examination and chart documentation.

Smoking has been, in some texts, linked to pulmonary embolism. I would suggest to you that smoking is more of a disease of the coronary arteries and the cerebral arteries, so patients who smoke do have a higher incidence of stroke and heart attack, but not as much venous disease such as DVT or pulmonary embolism. There was one study in patients who smoked and on birth control pills that seemed to have a higher incidence of venous disease.

The best diagnostic test to rule out pulmonary embolism is

a chest CAT scan with contrast. A ventilation perfusion scan (V-Q scan) is a poor test to diagnose pulmonary embolism. It is a nuclear study that looks at the perfusion of the lungs after ventilation of the lungs. With nuclear material, there is gross variation between a radiologist and the read of these, and therefore has been suggested by experts that a V-Q scan should be about equal to your clinical suspicion. So, if you have someone who just got off a plane ride, just had knee surgery, have a history of cancer and mother had a blood clot, and now presents with a swollen leg and shortness of breath, your clinical suspicion that the patient has pulmonary embolism should be extremely high. If the V-Q scan comes in at moderate probability, you really need to throw that and trust your suspicion as a clinician.

A lab test called a D-Dimer is a split fibrin product. This is going to be elevated when there is blood clotting in the body. This is a very un-sensitive test and of very low clinical utility. Studies that looked at the D-Dimer test suggest that if it is up, it tells us very little. If it is negative, it says there is not a pulmonary embolism. There is a lot of skepticism about this test among emergency room doctors and clinical care doctors. I do not know if I have ever seen a board-certified emergency room doctor order this. However, there are doctors who do put a lot of weight on the D-Dimer. If the D-Dimer is normal, it is not a pulmonary embolism. This has not been proven in literature. I find that I don't even order it because it does not help me much. If someone comes in as a high-risk patient for pulmonary embolism and their spiral CT scan is not conclusive, but their D-Dimer is negative, I am not sending that patient home. In a recent conversation with a boarded emergency physician, he felt if you had a patient with a low clinical suspicion of pulmonary embolism and a negative D-Dimer, be assured the patient does not have a PE.

Also in the diagnostic testing category for pulmonary

embolism is doppler of the legs. If someone comes in with a swollen leg and chest symptoms, and you are pretty sure this is pulmonary embolism, first of all, anticoagulate them sooner rather than later. If you give them an anticoagulant dose of Lovenox or place on Heparin drip even before sending them to radiology and they then go to radiology and have a bad outcome, there is nothing you could have done better for that patient. Under these circumstances, if you have a swollen leg and chest symptoms, you could very easily clinch the diagnosis by getting doppler of their legs, and that is a very quick, noninvasive test. If positive in the leg, they have at the very least a DVT that requires anticoagulation. The amount of time of anticoagulation will vary between whether it is truly a DVT. Some experts recommend anticoagulation for six months, versus a year for pulmonary embolism. The amount of time is really physician dependent and also dependent on what caused them to have the clot in the first place.

There are two ways to treat pulmonary embolism and/or DVT. That is with anticoagulation or inferior vena cava filter. I would say that approximately 19 out of 20 patients, or maybe 29 out of 30 patients, get anticoagulated where we will put them on Lovenox or Heparin and then switch them over the Coumadin for out-patient therapy. Patients who are at very high risk for bleeding such as people with brain tumors or history of anemia or peptic ulcer disease with occult blood positive stool, a vascular surgeon will go in through the femoral vein and put an inferior vena cava filter in. Some people call this an umbrella filter or a Greenfield filter. If a blood clot from the deep venous system of the legs goes upstream, it will get caught in this umbrella and not make its way to the lungs. Once again, the most important part of this diagnosis is clinical suspicion. You really need to keep sharp to look for pulmonary embolism.

In doing some chart reviews of patients who did have documented pulmonary embolism, I would like to describe the chart of a patient I had. Starting these are the timing intervals: She had a fever. She had a temperature of 100.3° and 101.2°. She was breathing fast at a rate of 42. She is a 49-year-old white female with a history of stroke two months ago and renal disease requiring a nephrectomy and had surgery pending. She presented with right shoulder pain and a cough that had a gradual onset starting yesterday. Patient states she had a cough that has been dry for the past two months. The patient states that prior to shoulder pain, there was an increased intensity in her cough.

I saw this lady in the emergency department actually two months prior for a CVA. She came in with right arm numbness and tingling, and we diagnosed her with stroke and I shipped her off to a bigger hospital. When I saw her this time, I asked how things went. She told me they had to remove a thrombus from her neck. As she described this, she was not talking about a carotid endarterectomy. She said that they actually had to do arterial surgery to take this blood clot out of her neck, which I thought was weird. Also, she said that they found out one of her kidneys was dead. I asked what that was from and she said they did not know but thought it may have been injured as a child. So, basically they are going to have to go in and do surgery on this kidney. So, going forth, when you look at the objective findings she had a temperature of 100.3°, respiratory rate that is up, but yet not in any kind of acute distress. So, she had positive right lower pleuritic chest pain. As my thoughts progressed on this patient, I started wondering if this could be pulmonary embolism and not infectious. I actually went back and asked a specific targeted question. But, on physical exam, her neck was supple with no jugular venous distention or bruit. Cardiovascular system was regular with S1/S2, no murmurs. Pulses were symmetrical upper and lower. On respiratory, she had splinting respirations with decreased breath sounds on the right, no rales or wheezes. Extremities had no edema. So, I started working her up, and when all was said and done, her EKG was normal sinus rhythm, no ischemia. Chest x-ray showed right lower lobe atelectasis. She had a white count of 15,000 with 4 bands. The rest of her chemistries looked fine, according to my medical logic.

Now, I was diagnosing with atelectasis and was concerned about pulmonary embolism or mass, and I worked her up for this. Now, this atelectasis I think was very tricky to see and was glad I had a two-view chest x-ray and a radiologist to look at it with me. When you review the radiology chapter under the germs that cause pneumonia, it is a bronchial pneumonia that causes atelectasis. Basically, these are germs that would infect the bronchia and cause the lung to collapse. I know it happens, but normally these patients look pretty sick because these germs are such as E. Coli or pseudomonas or staph or anaerobes. She did not look that toxically ill to me. She really did not look highly infected even though she had a white count and low-grade temperature. I am well aware (which will also be covered under the radiology chapter) that pulmonary embolism can present with atelectasis. It was with this information that I called her doctor and we did ship the patient off to a bigger hospital where they could more thoroughly work her up for pulmonary embolism, and it was called back later that night that this lady's lungs were filled with pulmonary embolism.

Now, I also documented Virchow's triad (and I do this on every patient with chest symptoms). I asked her about Virchow's triad; When she was in the hospital, was she at prolonged bedrest? She said they had her up walking every single day. I thought that she probably would not fall into the category of stasis. Was there damage to blood vessels? She said that they did not do any surgery on the lower extremities. What really got my attention was the blood clot in her left carotid and the fact that she had this necrotic kidney. It was with that information that made me question whether this patient could possibly have an undiagnosed hyper-coagulable state from a genetic predisposition. It made me think about whether there could be something going on in her body that caused her to have this thrombus in her neck and kill off her kidney. With this information, was it a long shot? Sure, it was a long shot, but as a mid-level provider, my job is to take all the information and give it to the physician, which I did. I called her doctor and gave him the information I had. If he would have said, "I see what you are saying, but I just want to send her home. Put her on antibiotics and send her home," I do not feel it would have been unreasonable. In this case, I think we got lucky.

The next case I want to talk about again illustrates the importance of risk factors and the importance of documentation. A 74-year-old white male presented with left lower chest pain for two days. He said that it was the same pain he had in the past when having pneumonia. It hurt more when he breathed. He did have chills the night before. He had a dry cough, no sputum. Vital signs were stable, no fever. Overall, clinically, he looked pretty good. However, I remember going back to my room and telling myself I would check some labs and a chest x-ray and started writing up the chart. His vital signs were stable, afebrile, 02 saturation of 97% on room air, no acute distress. Neck was supple. Cardiovascular showed regular rate and rhythm, no murmurs. Pulses +1 and +2 upper and lower. Lungs were clear with no rales or splinting. Chest wall pain was not reproducible. With the extremities, at first I wrote down no edema. Now, as I got information, up at the top on the right, I started documenting my cardiac risk factors and my Virchow's triad. He really did not have any cardiac risk factors. On Virchow's triad, I realized that I did not ask him this. So, I went back and asked whether he had any blood clots. He did not. Did he have any broken bones or injuries to the lower extremities? Now he states that he broke his ankle about eight weeks ago. Now I realized that my examination of his lower extremities was not very astute and went back and reexamined his legs.

I now realized that indeed his right lower extremity was bigger than the left. Therefore, under Virchow's triad I documented that he had had a lower extremity fracture and that his legs were disproportionate in size. His chest x-ray showed a left base opacity. He had a normal white count. With this, I called his doctor and said that this guy may very well have a DVT. The physician, who is a very good doctor, said that he thought this was probably pneumonia but to anticoagulate just in case and put him on antibiotics. If this were indeed a DVT and pulmonary embolism, it's an admission diagnosis. If it's a DVT and pneumonia yet the guy looks so good, you can still make an argument for admission, but this patient was anticoagulated and we discharged him home to be followed up by his own doctor the next day. The following day, as I talked to the doctor, they found this gentleman did indeed have a deep venous thrombosis and did require long-term anticoagulation and Coumadin. The doctor also suggested he had pneumonia as well which makes me concerned that possibly it was not a pneumonia but indeed a pulmonary embolism.

Those are two examples of how sizing a patient up for risk factors has saved my butt in the past. I cannot recommend it enough for you folks as providers.

The last letter in PAPPA is A for aortic dissection. So, PAPPA again is pericarditis, acute coronary syndrome, pneumothorax, pulmonary embolism and A is aortic dissection. This is not an abdominal aortic dissection. It is a thoracic aortic dissection where blood dissects through the aorta. Usually this is seen in older patients with long-standing history of hypertension or connective tissue disease. What happens is, as the vessel pops and rips through the intima, it causes extreme pain. Typically it radiates to the back and patients will describe it as a ripping or tearing sensation. Once that has occurred, the pain seems to subside, and the dissection between the vessel is relatively painless, so these people have a severe, agonizing episode of chest pain (a 10 out of 10 chest pain, radiating to the back) and then the pain seems to subside. That is what will have them present to the emergency room. More times than not, you will think this is an acute coronary syndrome. The initial diagnosis should be made from a chest x-ray with a high degree of clinical suspicion thinking that this could be a thoracic aneurysm. When diagnosing a thorasic aneurysm, the mainstay is a widened mediastinum. Although there is no exact criteria to evaluate whether the mediastinum is wide or not. It has been suggested that 8 cm is considered wide. If you hold your pager up to the mediastinum and if the mediastinum is bigger than your pager, it suggests that it is indeed enlarged and you should do more of a work up with a CAT scan or echocardiogram, for aortic aneurysm.

From a physical exam perspective, you really want to document symmetrical pulses of the upper and lower extremities. If you want more of an objective reading, have the nurse do blood pressures in both arms. A gross discrepancy could suggest that blood is being shunted into this aneurysm and not going to the one arm. Also, you want to document that there has been no murmur. Now, what happens is when you have a thoracic aneurysm and the intima starts getting dissected away, normally the dissection is distal. But, when the dissection is proximal, it will go to the aortic valve and make the valve incompetent so will have a new diastolic murmur of aortic insufficiency. The dissection of the intima can cause a flap of the intima to occlude the circumflex artery. What will happen in this circumstance is a patient will come in with the terrible chest pain and with EKG will appear just like a left lateral wall acute myocardial infarction. If you push thrombolytics it would be catastrophic.

Two different patients now come to mind. I was at a peer review where a physician had a patient come in with acute myocardial infarction pattern and ordered thrombolytics. The only reason he did not push the thrombolytics was because it took a while to get there from the pharmacy. The lab technician then came over with test results showing a very ominous appearing mediastinum that did prove to be a thoracic aortic dissection. He admitted right at peer review that if the thrombolytics would have been there, he would have pushed them, but the patient would have died.

The next patient was an elderly gentleman I saw when working as an in-patient house officer. He was admitted through the emergency department with an episode of chest pain. I evaluated him, talked to him and his wife, and it was made very clear that some major catastrophic event took place. They were eating dinner when he got this severe chest pain and broke out into a sweat. The wife said he got pale and she felt he was going to die. So, they came into the emergency department. His work up was relatively non-diagnostic, but we admitted him to rule out acute coronary syndrome. I actually gave him the heparin talk stating that we needed to thin the blood to keep his heart protected. But, in the process of doing my paperwork, I would always have a special spot where I would put down the medications that were given in the emergency room. They had given him a little bit of nitroglycerin. Of concern to me was that they had also given him about a liter's worth of I.V. fluids for blood pressure support because his blood pressure, systolically, was about 90.

When I talked with the patient, asking how his blood pressure was normally, he said it was 120/80, which got my attention. He was one of those proactive people who stayed very involved in his own health care. I realized on his physical exam that his 02 saturation was in the low 90s and had rales in the left base. Something weird was going on here. I went back and looked at the chest x-ray myself, now using pretest probability to saying that it just did not look right. The mediastinum did indeed look wide. I brought back the emergency physician who did not seem to think that was the case, but then I showed it to another emergency room physician who thought it looked quite ominous. We did go ahead and scan this gentleman.

At 3 in the morning we pushed over the CAT scanner. I was feeling a bit embarrassed that I was causing a ruckus and I remember thinking that I possibly was going overboard. But, we scanned him. I went back and started admitting other patients. An hour later we got the phone call that this patient did indeed have a Type 1 thoracic aneurysm that was dissecting. This patient immediately went to the ICU and then was shipped to cardiothoracic surgery. I was told later that the patient did quite well.

Thoracic aneurysms come in two different flavors, Type 1 or Type 2. Type 1 means that the aneurysm dissection starts right at the base of the aortic valve and goes distal. Type 2 starts at the arch of the aorta and goes downstream. Type 2 aortic dissections are more medically manageable and Type 1 are managed by a cardiothoracic surgeon. We should defer judgment with both Type 1 and Type 2 to the cardiothoracic surgeon.

When we talk about other causes of chest pain or second tier causes of chest pain, we can talk about gastrointestinal, musculoskeletal, psychiatric, viral, and abdominal symptoms that can cause chest symptoms. But once again, always before ruling out or ruling in second tier causes of chest pain, you have to rule out PAPPA. A gastrointestinal issue could suggest peptic ulcer disease. These are people who have an ulcer that perforates either in the stomach or in the duodenum. You really want to look for a history of NSAID use or history of H. Pylori or even just a history of peptic ulcer disease. If they have it, you want to determine how they have a history of it. Do they have a history of endoscopy? What did they find?

Boerhaave's syndrome is basically a rupture of the esophagus. It typically happens with massive amounts of retching and vomiting. These people present as very sick and can look like they are going to die, similar to someone with acute myocardial infarction or a pulmonary embolism. The fact that they had this tremendous amount of retching before this pain came on is a key element in the history. I do not consider Boerhaave's in the PAPPA mnemonic because the history really is pretty suggestive and will point you in the right direction. The less intense version of Boerhaave's is a Mallory-Weiss tear. This is more of a minor tearing of the esophagus from retching. This can happen to someone who has vomited multiple times after a night of drinking, or can occur with hyperemesis gravidarum or in a patient who is ill from chemotherapy. If they come in with a little bit of blood in their emesis, it is really no big deal; just treat the emesis. As a new graduate, I was not sure if Mallory-Weiss was a call the surgeon in the middle of the night condition, and it really is not.

Any patient who has a gastrointestinal bleed needs to have a nasogastric tube. You need to determine whether this bleeding is upper GI, meaning the ligament of Treitz, or, is it south of the ligament of Treitz. The gastroenterologist or whoever is going to do the endoscopy really needs to know that. If someone comes in with bright red stool, it suggests bleeding that is very close to the anal sphincter as from diverticulum or hemorrhoids. Black stool is cause for more concern. It has actually traveled through the gastrointestinal tract and has been digested, that is why it comes out black. So, it is the black stool that you really need to place a nasogastric for and see if you are getting blood out of the stomach. If you get coffee ground emesis from the stomach, you know that the bleeding is north of the ligament of Treitz. The concern here is if you flush the stomach and evacuate all that coffee ground emesis, you need to flush the stomach with water and keep bringing the aspirate out. If the aspirate coming out of the stomach is tinged red or bloody reddish, you know that there is continual bleeding going on and this is more of a surgical urgency than someone you flush and it remains clear. If someone has gastrointestinal bleeding, you put a nasogastric tube in and get gastric aspirate out with no blood, you can take the nasogastric tube out because you know the bleeding is more distal to the pyloric sphincter. In anybody with gastrointestinal bleeding, you really need to give either a proton pump inhibitor or an H2 blocker I.V.

You can never go wrong with reading a gastrointestinal bleeder very similar to a trauma patient, an ectopic pregnancy patient, or a patient with abdominal aortic aneurysm that is bleeding. Immediately give two large I.V.s to give blood or I.V. fluids if needed, a Foley catheter, and get someone smarter than you into the loop. Clinically, I have seen patients with upper gastrointestinal bleeds or lower gastrointestinal bleeds who lost so much blood orally or rectally that the amount was shocking. I have seen people die right in front of me from gastrointestinal bleeding, and the room was just covered with blood. You have to respect gastrointestinal bleeding and know that if an ulcer pops, the person can die right in front of you, and there is nothing you can do.

Patients with cirrhosis are a land mine for gastrointestinal bleeding. These are chronic alcoholics who have cirrhosis and have a tendency for esophageal varices. These are veins in the distal lower esophagus, and if that vein pops, they are going to die because they are going to bleed out right in front of you. It's these people with cirrhosis or history of being a heavy alcoholic that have upper gastrointestinal bleeding that would never place a nasogastric tube in. If they are bleeding, you just don't do it because as you are passing a nasogastric tube and you pop that esophageal variceal, they are going to die right in front of you. It is the cirrhotic patients who also have problems with coagulation. Factors 2, 7, 9 and 10 are produced in the liver and someone with cirrhosis and decreased physiology of the liver has blood will not clot like it should. Actually, their PT/INR will be high, so they are more prone to bleed just because of the coagulopathy and that esophageal variceal that you could nick with the NG tube. On this same note, with patients who have had gastric bypass surgery, be very hesitant to place the NG tube without talking to their surgeon. And, from the trauma literature, we want to be very careful placing a nasogastric tube in someone with a facial fracture or facial injury. There have been case reports of trying to place a nasogastric tube in a patient with basal skull fracture, and the nasogastric tube actually going up into their brain. I believe this to be quite a rare occurrence, but it is discouraged by the Advanced Trauma Life Support literature.

From a musculoskeletal perspective, you know costochondritis, which can be easily producible with palpation and pleuritic in nature, typically happens in younger folks. Musculoskeletal issues, without question, can cause chest pain, but we want to entertain this possibility only after we rule out the more serious ones.

Patients with a sensation of anxiety or psychiatric disease can manifest symptoms through chest pain. I believe it is not necessarily that these people intentionally try to mislead the system. I really believe that their body thinks they have chest pain and come in with these symptoms. If a provider takes a strong line saying the patient is just faking, the patient is going to be defensive and can cause quite a stink, saying you are an incompetent provider.

When in the Marine Corps, I was active in Desert Storm. When I got back from Desert Storm, I knew I had only a couple of months before being discharged from the Corps. We spent a month of leisure time, very soft time, until we got back to full Marine Corps infantry training. Part of this training had to do with putting a full combat pack on and walking for an extended period of time such as 14, 16, 18, 20 miles. Typically this was only done on Friday because the body is so broken down after carrying 60 pounds for 16 miles that you need all weekend to recover. If they had done this on Monday during the training week, the troops would be useless for any kind of physical training the rest of the week. Knowing I was going to get out of the Marine Corps and start college in a couple of months, these full combat humps made me feel very discouraged. Now, I know I was having problems with my back, which, in hindsight, I would describe as a mild inconvenience. My concern was that these full combat load humps were going to cause my back to have severe problems, and I would seek medical attention and be very hesitant about pushing my back before I had a medical evaluation by a specialist.

When I look back at this, now that I am a medical provider, I could see that I had tremendous secondary gain by exacerbating my back injury. I do not think it was a cognizant decision. I did not sit in my room one night saying that I would make my back hurt more to get out of these humps. I feel that my symptoms were magnified because of the secondary gain and I do think that happens in patient care. I know it happens in patient care in the emergency room. It happens all the time when a parent comes in and exacerbates the symptoms the child is having who is sick and coughing, and they state that the child has not eaten or drank in two days. But, the child has wet tears, and it is very clear that the child has been drinking something or would not be having wet tears. So, what I am saying is that psychiatric disease definitely plays a component in maladies.

There is a psychiatric component in every patient and their illness. I am an emergency room provider making good money at work, and if I sprain my ankle it may be different than the nursing aide who sprains her ankle. It would be different if a hospital executive sprains his ankle. It would be different for you, as a medical provider, reading this book now. We all have different psychological reactions to maladies. We could all have the exact same injury, but I know if I miss work, I am going to have to use vacation time, so I am going to wrap my ankle with an ace wrap, use Motrin and tough it out. The nursing aide who may have a sprained ankle would possibly find being off work for a couple of days quite beneficial. So, just understand that anxiety and psychiatric components play a part in every malady we see.

It is also possible to have a viral cause of second tier chest pain. An example of this is herpes zoster, which typically follows a very particular dermatome. A patient may present with chest-like symptoms even before the rash appears. One of the ways you can identify this is, with very light fingers, touch the area that is sore. If they have significant symptoms from very soft finger touch, that should lead you down the road to thinking this may be herpes zoster that has not presented with a rash as of yet.

Abdominal pain such as cholelithiasis or pancreatitis can also present with symptoms that look like chest etiology. I know there are case reports of death from someone who presented with chest pain from pancreatitis, was given thrombolytics and subsequently died from it. We will discuss cholelithiasis and pancreatitis more under liver functions. Lastly, before you come upon a softer diagnosis of chest pain, you have to rule out the bad stuff. Always use the **"Who's your PAPPA"** mnemonic. Your career depends on it, and lives depend on it.

P	**PERICARDITIS**
A	**ACUTE CORONARY SYNDROME**
P	**PNEUMOTHORAX**
P	**PULMONARY EMBOLISM**
A	**ANEURYSM**

CHAPTER 5

URINALYSIS

The urinalysis is a great, noninvasive test. You can get valuable information from a urinalysis, including a patient's serum glucose, their level of liver function, their nutritional status and how well they are digesting calories. You can also see how dehydrated the patient is. So, we will talk about all that and break down the urinalysis.

There are two different parts to the urinalysis. One is the dip or dipstick, and the other is a microscopic evaluation on a spun-down specimen. On the dipstick, there is glucose. The glucose will flag as +1 to +4. +1 means a small amount of glucose being spilled. +4 means a lot of glucose is being spilled. The threshold of spilled glucose in the urine is approximately 180 mg/dl meaning that if someone's blood sugars are at 200, they will pop positive on their dipstick. If their glucose is 140-150, they still are diabetic but will not pop positive on the dipstick. So, the magic number for glucose in the urine is 180. Therefore, you should never see positive glucose in the urine of any patient who is a non-diabetic.

Bilirubin and urobilinogen both, though in slightly different ways, look at the liver. If you dip someone's urine and it is positive for bilinogen or urobilinogen, you really need to do blood work to look at the red blood cells and liver functions. Now, bilirubin is a break down product of blood, and if someone is having hemolysis for whatever reason (their red blood cells are popping like balloons), that will spill a lot of bilinogen into the blood and thus be filtered and flagged positive in the urine. Urobilinogen has to do with the break down of bilinogen by microbes in the intestines. If someone is positive for urobilinogen and bilinogen, at the very least you need to do a CBC and comprehensive profile. Ketones suggest no or very low glycogen stores. These are patients who have been vomiting for a prolonged period of time, had poor p.o. intake, are on the Adkins diet or have some metabolic problem in the body that is producing an excessive amount of ketones (such as diabetic ketoacidosis). The bottom line is that these people who are ketone positive require calories. Their glycogen stores are gone so we need to get their glycogen stores back with I.V. fluids or with dextrose to make sure they are eating.

With diabetics and diabetic ketoacidosis, they need calories, but not in the form of giving them calories. We have to make the calories available to their cells. Someone who is in diabetic ketoacidosis has all sorts of calories in their blood stream. The problem is that they just cannot get them into the cells. These patients need insulin to get the calories. A non-diabetic, such as someone with hyperemesis gravidarum, a pregnant woman who is throwing up intractably, we give I.V. dextrose solution to get the calories back in their body. Urine specific gravity is a really sensitive test that suggests whether a patient is dry or not. A high specific gravity suggests uro-concentration. The number we look for is pretty much 1.030 or 1.035. This shows very concentrated urine and suggests dehydration. As an ultra-endurance athlete who has done marathons, triathlons and iron man triathlons, I know the importance of hydration status. A crude gage that we use to make sure we are hydrated properly is that when we pee, we want to make sure our urine is relatively clear. So, once again we want to make sure we have dilute urine to suggest our body is hyperhydrated. On the other side of the coin, if you see someone with very yellow concentrated urine, that suggests dehydration. Also, if someone is taking vitamin supplements, the urine can appear quite fluorescent.

When a patient has blood in the urine, you need to look for kidney stone, renal disease, urinary tract infection, or if the patient is a female, you want to know if she is having her period. Some pearls about kidney stones. This can typically be diagnosed as you walk in to see the patient, who is probably writhing on the bed, they, bouncing around attempting to find a position of comfort. Understand that a colicky-like pain such as with a kidney stone, a gallstone or even labor contractions is when you have something that is too big to pass through the anatomical structure it is supposed to pass through. As the body attempts to use peristalsis to push the object forward and out, the body goes through immense pain. I have had many patients who have had both kidney stones and have had babies say they would much rather have a baby. Kidney stone pain is severe and debilitating. The cornerstone for diagnosis of a kidney stone is someone with that pain pattern that I described and blood in the urine. I do not recommend hanging your hat on that diagnosis based on the presentation. I would recommend checking blood work and doing diagnostic studies to document where the stone is, the size of the stone and to confirm the fact that your diagnosis is correct. I use a non-contrast CAT scan of the abdomen and pelvis. With a woman who is on her period, we really need to differentiate if there is blood in the urine, so you have to ask the nurse to catheterize. There is no way around this. With renal disease, if someone has a high BUN and creatinine and are flagging positive for blood and protein in the urine, you really need to do a 24-hour urine to see how much protein is in the urine. Urinary tract infections can also produce blood.

With regard to pH, I find very little correlation in the pH of urine to the pH of blood. I have tried to look this up and find some degree of correlation. Clinically, I have seen patients who were acidotic, but their urine not necessarily acidotic. So, the only way I can really figure to use pH clinically is with treatment of certain diseases such as tricyclic antidepressant overdoses or patients in rhabdomyolysis where we are going to use bicarbonate to alkalinize the blood and hopefully the urine, and therefore when we are using bicarbonate to alkalinize the blood, we will follow urine pH trying to keep the pH high. Protein in the urine is really used to diagnose renal disease and preeclampsia.

Nitrates are the smoking gun for infection. Nitrates are produced when pathological germs in the urine break down the cells. So, I would consider nitrates the smoking gun for urinary tract infections. You want to use that in conjunction with leukocytes. Leukocytes are your white blood cells, and a high leukocyte count suggests an immune response to germs that are present. The clinical scenario here is someone who comes in for an ankle sprain who has a urinalysis for a pregnancy test. Let's say that the test comes back nitrite positive, yet there is an insignificant number of white blood cells. If a patient does not have symptoms and they are nitrite positive, I recommend doing a culture of the urine, but not necessarily treating an asymptomatic patient just because the urine looks a bit funny. Wait to see what happens in a day or two when the urine sample comes back.

A pearl about evaluation of a patient for a urinary tract infection; a clean catch is imperative. A good, clean-catch urine means that the patient goes into the bathroom, wipes the meatus of the urethra off with an alcohol wipe, pees a little bit into the toilet, then gives you a urine sample from a midstream clean catch. A patient who did not clean themselves well and has a lot of epithelial cells in their urine and those epithelial cells will bring along with it bacteria such as white blood cells and red blood cells. In that case, highly contaminated urine can look like a urinary tract infection even though there is no true infection. I have looked at urine samples, filled with a skin cells, and felt certain that infection was present. After having the patient catheterized or giving a second sample with a good clean-catch, the second urine sample turned out to be completely normal. So, do not be fooled by an excessive number of epithelial cells suggesting a urinary tract infection. A common abbreviation in urines is TNTC which too numerous to count. So, if you see white blood cells too numerous to count, you can rest assured that they have a urinary tract infection.

A day later, when the culture and sensitivity report comes back, there is a magic number here. The culture and sensitivity will tell you basic gram stain and what germ it is, and that is helpful. But, we want to know the colony count. The colony count magic number is greater than 100,000. If a person has greater than 100,000 E. Coli, they have pathological germ in the urine that is in abundance. So, greater than 100,000, they indeed have a urinary tract infection. If you have a colony count that is 50-100,000 it is not enough. Or, 10-50,000, again that suggests an insignificant number of germs and you do not have to treat for infection. Greater than 100,000, that indeed suggests a urinary tract infection.

If someone has gastrointestinal bleeding or sepsis and the body is not perfusing well, it is critical to monitor for shock. Put in a Foley catheter and use an urometer to measure output. Less than 70 cc in a two-hour period in an adult means that these patients are becoming shocky. I have put Foley catheters in many patients I felt were septic or having a lot of gastrointestinal bleeding. Look at the urinary output every two hours. If the output is dropping from 200 cc in a two-hour period down to 100 cc and then again down to 70 cc, you know, with such a significant decrease in output, they are getting sick and knocking on death's door.

Now, when you put a Foley in someone, the body has a reservoir that is going to put out a certain amount of urine as soon as the Foley is inserted. That reservoir is your bladder, and we are not concerned about that 100-300cc amount of fluid. It is irrelevant to assessing the patient for shock so we throw that urine away. We want to know how much urine is being produced over a period of time. It is this ins and outs or I/O that surgeons are concerned with. So, for a PA who is doing rounds on a patient postoperatively, a surgeon wants to know the amount of fluid in versus the amount of fluid out. Normal urinary output for a patient is about ½ cc per kg per hour, so about 80 cc per kilogram, maybe 70 or 60 in someone who is more petite. In children, that is double so it is 1 cc per kg per hour in children.

Now, let's look at some key concepts in urine and renal disease. Acute renal failure means acute alteration in renal function. The exact criteria for acute renal failure is really not well defined, however, if there has been acute alteration in renal function, it suggests that the patient has acute decompensation. I have a low threshold to say that a patient is in acute renal failure, (Especially if they are in a metabolic acidosis, which we will talk about at a later time). In someone with elevated renal functions, it is critical to determine whether this is prerenal, renal, or postrenal. We cannot let this go. We cannot say they have increased renal functions and not address it in more detail. Therefore, if someone is to be evaluated for renal disease, we need to start with a urinalysis, then move to BUN and creatinine and then an ultrasound of the kidneys. Understand that an EKG to a cardiologist is what the ultrasound is to a nephrologist. Do not send a patient to a nephrologist for a kidney work up without having had an ultrasound done. Renal failure can be classified as polyuric, oliguric or anuric which basically means that if someone is in renal failure, are they polyuric which means their kidneys do not filter but do make water and the patient can pee out urine. Oliguric means a middle amount. Anuric means that they just don't pee less than 100 cc per day. So, when I see a patient in the emergency room who has renal failure and is on hemodialysis, I will ask them if they make urine.

The most important question to ask a renal failure patient is how often they get dialysis and when they had it last. Typically, it is three times per week that they receive dialysis. If they have renal failure and are dialysis, ask when was their last dialysis. I would suggest that all patients who have hemodialysis are hyperkalemic and in congestive heart failure or have some degree of fluid retention, at varying degrees, based on their last dialysis. Also, these patients will be in metabolic acidosis from all of the acidic gook that is not being filtered. Again, that is relative to their last dialysis. So, hemodialysis patients chronically have an elevated sodium bicarbonate on their basic chemistry panel to compensate for the metabolic acidosis.

In discussion of renal insults that are common, ACE inhibitors and angiotensin respective blockers, you can expect about a 20% increase in creatinine. So, if the patient has a creatinine of 1.0 and you place them on an ACE inhibitor, you can expect that to go up to 1.1 or 1.2 after treatment. I.V. contrast from radiologic studies will potentially damage the kidneys, and this is particularly important in diabetics who are on Glucophage. The standard of care right now is that if a patient is on Glucophage and needs a contrast study such as an angiogram or a pulmonary embolism work up with a chest CAT scan with contrast, we would check their BUN and creatinine. If they are normal and on Glucophage, you would go ahead and do the study and hold the Glucophage for two days and then recheck their renal functions. If their renal functions are elevated such as with a creatinine of 2.0 and are on Glucophage, the study would be withheld until the patient is adequately hydrated so the creatinine comes down to an acceptable level before the test. If a patient has a high creatinine and is on Glucophage, and you need to do a contrast dye study, you really need to talk with the specialist before initiating care. Remember, the Glucophage is a buzzword of causing lactic acidosis, especially in patients with renal disease. Gentamycin, a high potency antibiotic, can cause renal disease, and anti-inflammatory medications or NSAIDs. NSAIDs are Motrin, Advil, ibuprofen, and Indocin. These medications affect the afferent arterials going into the glomerulus and cause them to be stressed. If you put any patient, (especially elderly) on anti-inflammatory medications, you have to be really concerned about their kidneys. If they have a mild degree of renal insufficiency, this can make their filtering much worse, increase their creatinine, and have them retain more fluid. An NSAID, can cause a patient to go into congestive heart failure. In my years of being a physician assistant and using the most potent medications in medication from paralytics (before rapid sequence intubation) to thrombolytics for people with acute coronary syndrome, I have not found a medication more troublesome or that has gotten me into more trouble than the anti-inflammatory.

Not only can these drugs affect the kidneys, they can cause peptic ulcer disease or irritate a peptic ulcer. Anti-inflammatories do not mix well with Coumadin. If a patient is on Coumadin and require an analgesic, I would recommend staying away from the NSAID class and going more to an opioid. Anti-inflammatories can have cross reactivity with aspirin allergies. So, if a patient says they have an aspirin allergy, you should not give them Motrin, Advil, ibuprofen or Toradol. Aspirin works great. It is a miracle medication for acute coronary syndrome. Anti-inflammatories do have an antiplatelet effect that makes aspirins not as effective. So, if a patient is on aspirin, which is working well to prevent them from having a heart attack or stroke, the introduction of anti-inflammatories would increase their risk of heart attack or stroke. You want to avoid using anti-inflammatories in people who have coronary artery disease and who are on aspirin.

Inflammatory medications are contraindicated in the third trimester of pregnancy. They say you can use this in the 1st and 2nd trimesters, yet is discouraged throughout the medical world. The theory is that the ductus arteriosis in fetal circulation is kept open by prostaglandins. Anti-inflammatories are anti-prostaglandins, and if a woman who is in her third trimester is given an anti-inflammatory (anti-prostaglandin) it could cause the ductus arteriosis to close and lead to fetal demise.

If a neonate is born and they have a patent ductus arteriosis, they actually use I.V. Indocin (anti-prostaglandin) to close it and improve circulation outside of the womb. On the flip side, if a neonate has a cardiac anomaly and a left to right shunt, typically about 7-10 days out, when that ductus arteriosis is closing, the babies go into shock. You always want to think sepsis. In any neonate who is turning crappy, there are 10 things that can cause it, and the first nine are shock. Shock. Shock. Shock. Shock. You want to treat with high-dose antibiotics. If this is found to be a true cardiac anomaly, and the ductus arteriosis is closing, we would actually give I.V. prostaglandins to keep it open until a pediatric thoracic surgeon can correct the problem.

In further discussion of renal disease, nephrotic syndrome and pyelonephritis are some important buzzwords to remember. Acute tubular necrosis is destruction of the tubular epithelial cells. This can be ischemic, from a shock state or nephrotoxins. Chronic renal failure, as we talked about, is basically renal disease with cronic high levels of creatinine. This can predispose a patient to requiring dialysis. Just as notable, if they have chronic renal disease or renal insufficiency, it is a condition that must be observed.

Hydronephrosis is a dilation of the renal pelvis and calices, seen commonly with obstruction such as kidney stones. Earlier in my career, I found it really concerning if someone had hydronephrosis or hydroureter meaning that the obstruction caused a blockage and stress in the ureter and kidney. Similar to the Mallory-Weiss tear, I was not sure how big of a deal that was until I actually talked to a urologist about it. The advice the urologist gave me was that if a patient has two functioning kidneys and two functioning ureters, you can tie a ureter in a knot for two weeks, come back two weeks later, untie the ureter and the kidney would do fine. I am not convinced that I would give an obstructive uropathy two weeks, but I now know that when someone presents with hydroureter or hydronephrosis, they can go a day or two without the problem being corrected.

Admission diagnosis/criteria for kidney stone includes intractable pain, intractable vomiting or a pyelonephritis with a kidney that is infected on top of the kidney stone. Do not ever hesitate to contact urology prior to making those decisions. We discussed the terrible pain that Nephrolithiasis or urolithiasis, or kidney stones, can cause. With these patients, you always want to strain their urine to see if you can get a piece of the stone to analyze. I would say that 9 out of 10 times it is a calcium stone and there is not much we can do with those. You want to educate the patient saying that if it is their first stone, 50% of the time they will have a second stone. If they have a second stone, you can say that they are going to have stones for the rest of their life; it's just how it is. In the rare incidence the stone is pyruvate or uric acid, there are specific treatments for those stones.

Nephrotic syndrome has to do with massive proteinuria meaning greater than 3-5 g per day, where the patient is actually peeing out their albumin and has a low serum albumin. When someone is in a low albumin state, they will have diffuse third spacing of fluid, and will have edema. They will have elevated lipids. Because they are peeing so much, they are peeing out their coagulation factors and will be in a hypercoagulable state. So, a buzzword of urinary issues is nephrotic syndrome.

Pyelonephritis has to do with kidney infections. Typically, we see this in young women. If a pregnant woman comes in with pyelonephritis, that is an admission diagnosis and we use very aggressive antibiotic therapy with a non-fluoroquinolone antibiotic. Remember fluoroquinolones will cause damage to the growing fetus. However, it has been my experience that if a young woman comes in, not pregnant, with a pyelonephritis, a temperature of a 103° and white blood cell count of 18,000, they do remarkably well in the emergency room if you give them a couple liters of fluid and I.V. antibiotics.

Willie Sutton was a bank robber in the early 1900s, and he was credited for the following saying. A reporter asked him, "Willie, why did you rob banks?" Willie said, "Because that's where the money is." So, where is the money when it comes to urinalysis? With urinary tract infections, you want to look for white blood cells and nitrates. If positive, do a culture and sensitivity. In kidney stones, we are looking for blood. With ketones, if the glucose is positive and greater than 180, you need to remember that treatment needs to be calories, either orally or with I.V. dextrose solution.

Remember that with urine, we can do a pregnancy test. A urine pregnancy test, a urine human chorionic gonadotropin) is just as sensitive and just as reliable as a blood test. So, if someone comes in saying they are pregnant, took a home test, which was positive, but just wanted to check it in the emergency room, it is really the same test. I would never recommend denying a woman who wants a pregnancy test in the emergency room, just do it. But, understand that the blood test may detect the HCG a bit earlier but is not more sensitive. As a side note, when would an HCG be positive in a male? The answer is testicular cancer. They would have a positive HCG such as Lance Armstrong. In his book, Lance stated that his HCG was positive and indeed high, and that was the marker for testicular tumor. From the urine, we can do urine toxicology screening. If we want to see if someone overdosed, even though they have very little role in acute management of overdoses and poisons, it can steer you in the direction if a patient is taking one of the more common recreational drugs.

You will hear commenting about glomerular filtration rate or basically the filtering ability of the kidneys. That is kind of an ideal measurement of how well the kidneys are filtering. A more clinically relevant rate to see how well they are filtering is creatinine clearance. There is a formula to calculate this, and this may be relevant if you are using specific drugs like Gentamycin or Vancomycin, but this book is not about formulas, and if you need to know the formula, I would refer you to a different text.

There has always been talk about dopamine and renal dose dopamine. Let me explain. Dopamine is a catecholamine or sympathomimetic that stimulates the sympathetic nervous system. It is suggested that dopamine has different physiologic responses at different doses. Between 2 and 5 mCg per minute, it dilates the renal arteries. When at 5-10 mCg, it is a positive ionatrope, making the heart beat stronger. At 10-20 mCg, it is a vasopressor and increases blood pressure. There has been the thought that if someone is septic or not getting good blood flow to the kidneys for whatever reason, low-dose dopamine may perfuse the kidneys better. This is really not as accurate as it looks in the textbooks. It has been my experience that nephrologists do not like renal dose dopamine and they think that actually vaso- constricts and deviates blood away from the kidney. I do not know of any literature to support this one way or the other.

It has been my experience as a nighttime house officer that if I had a patient with borderline blood pressure, despite adequate I.V. fluids, with a tremendous amount of peripheral vasodilation, typically from sepsis, and I had a tough time keeping their blood pressure up with I.V. fluids, I would want to go with dopamine. Now, on the floor in the hospital, I was not allowed to use dopamine at any higher dose than renal dose dopamine, meaning 2-5 mCg. If I needed it as a vasopressor, the patient was required to go to the ICU. I would run my renal dose dopamine as high as I could get away with and get some degree of pressure support to hopefully keep them on the floor where I could manage. If a patient got too sick, obviously I would move them to the unit, but I kind of felt it was failed medical management on my part if I had to move a patient to the ICU.

CHAPTER 6

ABDOMINAL LAB TESTS

First off, I want to talk about liver function tests, which are the AST and ALT, GGT, alkaline phosphatase, and bilirubin. AST stands for aspartate aminotransferase. ALT stands for alanine aminotransferase. GGT stands for gamma glutamyl transpeptidase. Alk phos stands for alkaline phosphatase.

When we have a patient with elevated LFTs, it is important for us to determine whether this is a hepatonecrotic pattern or cholestatic pattern. In the diagram on the next page, you realize that AST and ALT are contained within the hepatocytes. They are within the liver cells. The way to think about this is if liver cells are dying at a very rapid pace, you would have very high elevations of AST and ALT. In the ducts that run through the liver where bilirubin travels, the ducts are lined with GGT and alkaline phosphatase. So, when we evaluate a patient with abnormal LFTs, we want to know if it is hepatonecrotic pattern with massive amounts of AST and ALT with very mild elevations of bilirubin, alkaline phosphatase and GGT. On the other hand, when there is an obstructive problem, there is a massive backup of bilirubin and GGT and alkaline phosphatase when the AST and ALT are minimally elevated.

Some examples of hepatonecrotic patterns are seen with hepatitis, Tylenol overdose or any hepatotoxic drug. In cholestatic pattern, by far the most common is gallstone. If you have a gallstone that is stuck in the common bile duct, you will have significant elevations in total bilirubin and mild elevations in AST and ALT. I can say that clinically when it comes to liver functions, I really only care about AST, ALT and total bilirubin. If the GGT or alkaline phosphatase levels are up, that really is not as specific. Once again, I hang my hat on the AST and ALT and total bilirubin.

Another liver function test is LDH (lactic dehydrogenase). This is a very nonspecific enzyme found in the heart muscle. It also has isoenzymes similar to CPK, but I have never ordered them and never heard of them being ordered in my career. Serum albumin and protein are synthesized in the liver. Severe hypoalbumin states are seen in end-stage liver failure. This will cause third spacing of fluids.

Fluids are kept in check within their intravascular space by two major pressure systems. One is a hydrostatic pressure system and one is an osmotic pressure system. Hydrostatic basically means forward flow of water with the heart as the pump. So, hydrostatic pressure is basically water pressure from a pump. Osmotic pressure has to do with the solutes that are in blood, which keep balance between the three spaces in the body that hold fluid; the blood vessel, the cell or interstitium. The interstitium is basically in between cells. So, once again, fluid is held within one of three spaces, in the cell, outside the cell or in the blood vasculature. Fluid is constantly shifting back and forth based on the hydrostatic and oncotic pressure. Oncotic pressure is largely determined by sodium but is also determined by albumin. Patients with very low albumin states will go have diffuse swelling throughout their body, as seen in nephrotic syndrome, pancreatitis or people with chronic wasting away from malnutrition or liver failure. These patients can have tremendous swelling in their legs, and you can give them all the diuretics that you want, but the treatment is to increase osmolality and give serum albumin.

Prothrombintine and INR are clotting factors that are made in the liver (these are Factors II, VII, IX and X). The most critical lab value to evaluate hepatic physiology is the PT/INR. Someone could have elevations in their AST and ALT but still have a very well functioning liver. If the liver decides to quit, and doesn't want to work anymore, you will know that by the INR being high. These people will be prone to bleeding.

I recall a patient with cirrhosis who came in jaundice, kind of obtunded, not acting quite right, and the family was concerned. As I looked at the gentleman, he was clearly jaundice. He had yellow skin and had a degree of altered mental status. When I ran some lab work on him, I realized that his INR was approximately 3. Remember, normal reference range in someone who is not anti-coagulated is approximately 1. An INR of 3 means the blood is significantly thinned. His blood was so significantly thinned that his liver had almost completely stopped functioning. When I looked at his history, approximately six months before, this patient had an INR of about 1.2 or 1.3. This man had a INR of 3, so he was in fulminant liver failure and was going to die soon without a liver transplant. The patient was not a candidate for a liver transplant, and I had to discuss this with the family. He was admitted to the hospital and did pass away the following day.

Ammonia (NH3) is another evaluated liver function that, when elevated, indicates that the patient will become obtunded. They will become sleepy, and not act quite right. This is very similar to a patient who is hypercarbic from high levels of carbon dioxide. The treatment is lactulose. Lactulose will bring ammonia levels down until they become more alert and oriented. I have seen patients who have had liver insufficiency and elevated liver functions be on 3 times per day lactulose just to keep the ammonia level down. One time I had a patient come in to the emergency room who said she wanted to have her ammonia level checked. When I asked why, she said she thought she had ammonia. When I asked what made her think that, she said she was coughing and had a fever, so she thought she had ammonia. I found that quite silly because it became clear to me that she meant pneumonia not ammonia.

As an FYI, here are some liver function basic evaluation patterns of the AST and ALT. With hepatitis or viral hepatitis, you would expect AST and ALT to be about 200 times normal.

Remember that AST and ALT normally is about 50. When we discussed normal patterns of AST and ALT, we normally talk about times normal. So, when you have an AST and ALT that are four times normal, you are looking at an AST and ALT of approximately 200. Someone who has chronic cirrhosis from alcoholism, you are looking at AST and ALT of about 100 to 400. With cirrhosis with a completely cirrhotic liver, you can have mild to no elevation because the liver is shot. Biliary cirrhosis or obstruction, you would expect a mild elevation in the AST and ALT of approximately 200.

Let's now focus on pancreatic enzymes and amylase and lipase. Lipase is the smoking gun of pancreatitis. If it is elevated, it is a clear indicator of pancreatitis. Nowhere else in the body is lipase secreted other than the pancreas. Amylase is less sensitive and can be secreted for other reasons other than for pancreatitis. Amylase is indeed made in the pancreas but is also made in the salivary gland in the mouth. In a patient who presents with pancreatitis, there are really two main causes. One is EtOH, so the patient is a chronic drinker. The second is gallstones. A tertiary reason could be triglycerides, but that is a whole lot less common. Pancreatitis presents with severe epigastric pain that radiates to the back. If a patient has pain that radiates to the back, a couple buzzwords are aneurysm and pericarditis.

If you have a patient with pain that radiates to the back, the big issues you need to be concerned with are pancreatitis, aneurysm or pericarditis. These patients typically present with excessive vomiting. To work up these patients from an historic perspective, you really want to get a good history for fatty food intolerance or what is called the four F's, which are common with gallbladder disease. They are fat, female, fertile and forty. Those seem to go together. Normally, it is a woman who is 40 years old and relatively obese who presents with gallbladder disease. Demerol and morphine are both okay to use for pancreatitis. There is older literature that suggests

Demerol is much better, and morphine is not as good. Some of the older surgeons still believe that, that if you give morphine it can cause excessive contraction of the sphincter of Oddi and make patients worse. Of interest is that these studies were done on the biliary tract of cat models. From veterinarian literature, it was realized that the biliary tract of cat models is not very similar to those of humans. So, it was redone on the biliary system of opossum models, and it was found that both contract the sphincter of Oddi a bit, but to a negligible degree between the two so Demerol and morphine are both okay. The treatment of pancreatitis is pain control, bowel rest and I.V. fluids. This is an admission diagnosis. They get pain control, are not allowed to eat anything and receive aggressive I.V. fluids. A nasogastric tube is not mandatory, but if the patient is having excessive vomiting, you should go ahead with one. These patients do require a right upper quadrant ultrasound looking for obstruction of the sphincter of Oddi.

Ranson's criteria is a criteria used to prognosticate how patients will do. High level of Ranson's criteria means that they have a high incidence of doing bad things, when a lower criteria means that they will most likely do well. The mnemonic is **GALL BOTCH**. G is glucose greater than 200. A is age greater than 55. L is leukocytosis. L is liver function tests that are elevated. And at 24 hours, the mnemonic is BOTCH where BUN is elevated which suggests third spacing of fluid. O is decreased oxygen. T is more specifically third spacing fluid where you are going to look at the Is and Os. C is calcium which means their calcium will drop. H suggests a decreased hematocrit where they are becoming increasingly edemic. Why would a patient become hypocalcemic with pancreatitis? There is a theory of saponification, which means that as the patient becomes sicker, the pancreas will actually form soap-like crystals of calcium in the pancreas. In a patient with chronic pancreatitis, we can actually see the calcium density on the pancreas on a plain-film radiograph.

G	**GLUCOSE GREATER THAN 200**
A	**AGE GREATER THAN 55**
L	**LEUKOCYTOSIS**
L	**LIVER FUCNTION TESTS ELEVATED**
B	**BUN IS ELEVATED**
O	**DECREASED OXYGEN**
T	**THIRD SPACING OF FLUID**
C	**CALCIUM**
H	**HEMOCRIT DECREASED (EDEMIC)**

Now let's focus on how to work up abdominal pain. We will break it down into the right upper quadrant and left upper quadrant, then go on to discuss the left lower quadrant, and the right lower quadrant. With right upper quadrant abdominal pain, you always need to be concerned about chest pathology. Do not get burned for right upper quadrant pain and think it is definitely in the stomach. It still could be pulmonary or cardiac. I do recall a young man who came in with right upper quadrant abdominal pain. I worked him up intensely thinking that it possibly was gallbladder in nature. He did have a history of a pneumothorax, so I paid very close attention to the lung thinking this could be a spontaneous pneumothorax or a pulmonary embolism, but most likely I thought it was biliary. With this patient, I was very close to discharging him for an out-patient ultrasound and work up of biliary disease, when at the last minute I did not think it felt right or seem right. I did transfer him to a bigger hospital just to figure out later that he did indeed have a pneumothorax that I was unable to pick up on his inspiratory and expiratory films. So, anybody with upper quadrant abdominal pain, do not get burned and forget about your life-threatening chest symptoms.

With chest symptoms ruled out, some buzzwords of gallbladder disease are fatty food intolerance and the four Fs and symptoms that occur at night. During the daytime, a patient sits upright so the stones will be lying in the inferior portion of the gallbladder. When the patient lies down at night, those stones actually go more posterior because of the bile that is in the gallbladder and gravity. In the posterior position, the gallbladder puts those stones closer to the duct, and at nighttime the stone is more prone to go into the duct and wake a patient up with severe pain. To remedy this, we would suggest sleeping with the head of the bed elevated or sleeping on pillows, once again using gravity to keep the stones away from the duct and not eating 3-4 hours before bed, in ordr to keep the gallbladder more calm at night.

The last buzzword of gallbladder disease is Murphy's sign. Murphy's sign has to do with palpating the right upper quadrant, and when the patient takes a deep breath it hurts. The physiology behind it is that you are taking the gallbladder and pushing it into the liver. When the patient takes a deep breath, it pushes on the diaphragm, pushes on the liver and pushes the gallbladder into your hand. Does it hurt when the patient takes a deep a breath, or do they splint when taking a deep breath? That would mean a positive Murphy's sign.

You can have someone with gallbladder disease who doesn't have stones, but this is less common. These patients can have an angry gallbladder that does not like to function even though there is no stone in there. This is a patient who presents with classic fatty food intolerance, right upper quadrant pain, but has a normal ultrasound. A surgeon will typically send the patient for a HIDA scan. This is a nuclear study where a patient will be injected with nuclear contrast that goes into the gallbladder and then they would be given CCK, which stands for cholecystokinin. This is a hormone that is secreted that causes the gallbladder to contract. So, this HIDA scan is done, and they receive the CCK. They watch the gallbladder contract, and if it does not contracting normally, the diagnosis is acalculi gallbladder disease. The patient will go on to have surgery.

Also in the right upper quadrant, we want to look at the liver, so we are going to look at liver functions, bilirubin, amylase and lipase, again ruling out pancreatitis. To rule out someone with liver disease, you want to look for food that they have recently ingested, looking more for Hepatitis A. Hepatitis A is basically just a fancy food poisoning. There are a significant number of people in modern cities who are positive for Hepatitis A and they might not even know. They might have said that they remember a couple of years ago they had really bad food poisoning. That very well could have been exposure to Hepatitis A. There are immunizations against Hepatitis A if you are going to a foreign country. Hepatitis A is a fecal oral issue and has to do with poor sanitary conditions in the food that is being prepared.

You want to look for past blood exposures to rule out hepatitis such as contaminated needles, sharing needles, multiple sex partners or blood transfusions before really starting to screen for hepatitis and HIV. Also, you want to look for excessive alcohol intake. Lastly, pancreatitis can present with right upper quadrant pain. Normally, it is epigastric pain so kind of in the middle between the right and left upper quadrants. With pancreatitis, you want to look for gallstones, want to get a good history, check and evaluate the patient's triglycerides. With pancreatitis, as we talked about, you want to assess Ranson's criteria. Courvoisier's law has to do with a palpable pancreas, jaundice with no pain. If you have a patient who presents with yellow skin, yet no pain, according to Courvoisier's law, you have to assume that is cancer of the head of the pancreas or of the biliary tree until proven otherwise.

Now looking at the left upper quadrant, we must rule out a life-threatening pathology such as myocardial infarction or pulmonary embolism. Very rarely have I found this to be of significant pathology in the left upper quadrant. Normally, you have to look at the stomach or peptic ulcer disease and really the mainstay of treatment here is a GI cocktail. Give them a GI cocktail, and the mnemonic I use is DMV where D is Donnatal, M is Maalox and V is viscus lidocaine. Donnatal is 10 cc, Maalox is 30 cc and Lidocaine is 10 cc. You give this to the patient and monitor to see how well that worked. If it really worked and you are confident it's peptic ulcer disease, you would put them either on proton pump inhibitor or H2 blocker. I cannot stress enough that therapeutic challenge is never diagnostic. So, if you give a patient a GI cocktail and they feel better, it is suggested it is their stomach but you cannot rule out cardiac based on positive response to a GI cocktail. With pain in the middle of the stomach, be concerned about an abdominal aortic aneurysm (AAA). The buzzword there is 5 cm. What happens is if a patient has an aneurysm that hits 5 cm, they have a tendency to progress very quickly after that. So, people with a AAA of 5 cm, that is when a surgeon would talk to them about having surgery. Centralized or generalized abdominal pain can also be seen with early appendicitis or just a bowel obstruction, where there is no specific place of pain.

In the right lower quadrant, the hot word is appendicitis. Typically, this presents with a vague epigastric-like umbilical pain that radiates to the right lower quadrant. Almost always, they will be anorexic, meaning they will not be hungry, and they will actually be repulsed by food. It is kind of like having a bad hangover (not that I have ever had one) and someone asks if you want pork chops. You just cannot possibly eat. That is a very common response in patients with appendicitis. Typically, they have a fever. Typically, they have leukocytosis. A CAT scan is the most helpful test, even though there is no perfect test for appendicitis. The patient really needs to be aware of this. A surgeon can go in to do an appendectomy only to find a normal appearing appendix. I can say in my experiences, appendicitis is indeed a great masquerader. I have seen people I was absolutely sure did not have appendicitis, have a positive CAT scan, go into the operating room and have an infected appendix. So, it is indeed a great masquerader.

The location of the appendix can vary. When someone has a retrocecal appendix, it means the appendix is a lot more posterior. In pregnant women, the gravid uterus will push the appendix up into the right upper quadrant. So, once again appendicitis is a great masquerader. With belly pain and right lower quadrant pain, these people have a low threshold to work up for appendicitis.

Some buzzwords are McBurney's point and Rovsing sign. McBurney's point is the area right between the umbilicus and the right ileac crest. You draw a line, and right in the middle of that line, that is where McBurney's point is. Rovsing sign when you palpitate the left lower quadrant, but the patient feels pain in the right lower quadrant. Psoas sign is flexion of the psoas muscle by extending the leg at the hip, and if this causes right lower quadrant pain, they have a positive psoas sign. Obturator sign is where you flex at the waist and at the knee and rotate the knee laterally. If that is positive, that stimulates the obturator muscle. If the obturator muscle is touching the appendix, that would cause pain as well. As much as they are not very specific, these are buzzwords of appendicitis. Remember that the right lower quadrant can also give you pyelonephritis or kidney stone which we talked about, and you want to do a urine sample looking for blood and white blood cells.

In the lower left quadrant, by far the most common issue is diverticulitis, especially in older folks. You want to look on the left for very similar symptoms to appendicitis on the right. You want to look for fever, and white blood cell count and do not hesitate to do a CAT scan looking for abscess formation or perforation.

There are some general rules about the work up of abdominal pain. All women are pregnant until proven otherwise. If I have a female who comes into the emergency room with belly pain, a nurse should be on automatic pilot to do a urinalysis and a pregnancy test before I even see the patient. If I see her and those tests are not done yet, they are just going to wait longer. I would rather come out and have that information available to me before going into the room. Once again, all women are pregnant until proven otherwise. Ectopic pregnancies kill young healthy women and if an ectopic pregnancy pops, they will bleed so much into their belly that they can die in a matter of minutes. Ectopic pregnancy is an obstetrical emergency. Positive HCG, progressive belly pain, they need an emergent ultrasound or emergent obstetrical evaluation. Bowel obstructions, whether it is small bowel or large bowel, will be covered more under radiology and the evaluation of abdominal films. These patients need I.V. fluids and nasogastric tube.

CHAPTER 7

COAGULATION

"TO BLEED OR NOT TO BLEED, THAT IS THE QUESTION"

Two things are needed to stop bleeding. One is a platelet plug and the second is a fibrin clot. These need to be thought of as completely separate entities even though the end product is hemostasis. Let's first talk about the platelet plug. Now, there are two main problems with platelets, either a decreased number or bad (broken) platelets that have poor function. There are two tests that we need to evaluate for platelet function. One is the platelet count as seen on the red blood cell count. So, we are looking at the absolute number, or we are looking at a test called the bleeding time. When a platelet count is decreased, this is known as thrombocytopenia. This occurs if there is a problem in the bone marrow such as decreased production of platelets from malignancies, and is commonly seen in chemotherapy that suppresses bone marrow. Thrombocytopenia can also occur from a hyperactive spleen (where the only potential solution is a splenectomy) or from idiopathic thrombocytopenia, which can appear in a child after a viral syndrome; the treatment is steroid removal immunoglobulin or spleen removal.

When I was in my pediatric rotation, which was actually my first rotation as a physician assistant student, I remember seeing a young child for a well child visit, and when the physician, who was a bit older with a beard, came in, the child was quite afraid of him and the mother said he looked like the boy's father. When the doctor examined the child, the child had a number of bruises especially on his lower legs. I was quite upset by this thinking this was a very clear case of child abuse and that the father was beating the child. The doctor sent him off for blood work, and I was quite upset with the physician and wondered aloud how he could not see that this was clearly a case of child abuse. Well, the blood work came back, and this child had idiopathic thrombocytopenia. The bruises were not from child abuse. A red flag is to think sepsis when you have unexplained thrombo-cytopenia, especially with children. With platelet counts lower than 50,000, you can get increased bleeding status post trauma. If you have platelet counts of less than 20,000, you can have increased spontaneous bleeding. When I used to cover the hematology / oncology floor, we would transfuse patients when they got below 10,000.

The bleeding time test is basically a small incision, or a very uniform little abrasion in the skin made by a spring-loaded apparatus. The lab will blot that area until the bleeding stops. I have maybe ordered the test once or twice in my career. It is pretty rare. The most common reason why platelets would not clot well is if someone takes aspirin and their blood is a little bit thin. Or uremia. Hypothermia can do this as well.

Remember that a platelet lives in the body for seven days, and when you take an aspirin this completely deactivates all platelets that are in the body. I will not discuss coagulopathies here such as Von Willebrand's or hemophilia. But, I do want to talk about medications that affect the platelets. The most common one by far is aspirin. The dose can vary between 81 mg to 1,000 mg daily. Plavix is typically 75 mg once per day, and has been used with success in people with known coronary artery disease or atherosclerotic disease such as a past myocardial infarction or stroke. Glycoprotein 2B and 3A inhibitors are used for unstable angina. It is kind of like a fancy IV aspirin.

In discussing formation of the clot as we learned in PA school, there are two basic pathways, the intrinsic and extrinsic pathway, and it is not clinically relevant to know all the factors in each pathway. Just be aware that it exists and is quite complicated. If you become a hematology / oncology provider, this may be more important, especially if you are dealing with hemophiliacs. Note that the intrinsic pathway, which is monitored by the partial thromboplastin time, or the PTT, is thinned and altered with the heparin drip. When it is the extrinsic pathway that is followed by the prothrombin time or the INR, that is altered by Coumadin. Think of a small country where there was going to be a war because a military unit threw a coup. They were concerned because it might cause an international incident, and these guys really had to train hard and do a lot of physical therapy. Warfarin, Coumadin, international ratio or INR and prothrombin; if you want to go a step further, you can say extrinsic pathway is that they had to exercise outside. Coumadin, Warfarin, international ratio, PT or prothrombin time, and extrinsic pathway are the important things to remember here. The INR is basically a standardized test of the prothrombin time, used to monitor Coumadin. The concern is that Coumadin thins the blood and is a pretty dangerous medication if the patient's blood becomes too thin.

Let's say grandma lives in Florida but comes to New York for the summer. She will go to two different labs to have her blood drawn to see how thin it is. Coumadin users normally get their blood checked once per month. If the tests are varied between Florida and New York, keeping the patient balanced therapeutically may be tricky. INR is a uniform way to calculate how thin someone's blood is, and the test is standardized from lab to lab.

Coagulation factors 2, 7, 9 and 10 are made in the liver. People in liver failure will have a coagulopathy and their PT/INR will be quite high. When this occurs, know that the liver is pretty much shot.

Patients with platelet disorders typically have superficial, light bleeding like petechia on the skin, spontaneous bleeding in the oral mucosa, gastrointestinal tract or genitourinary tract.

Platelet disorders can also cause a patient to void blood or have blood in the stool, or have spontaneous bleeding after trauma. Coagulation disorders normally have deep bleeding like deep bruises in their muscles or hemarthrosis in joints. These people typically have delayed bleeding after trauma such that someone who has a laceration, the first thing that is going to make the bleeding stop is the platelet plug, and then the fibrin clot forms after it.

How do we fix a coagulation problem? Well, if it is a platelet problem, we decrease number. If they have bad platelets, we give a platelet transfusion. Normally 6-8 units of platelets can be given every 6-8 hours. That is by far the less common cause of bleeding problems. The most common is a patient who is on Coumadin and, for some reason, the INR has gone extremely high. This can be due to medications or the patient accidentally taking too much. We have three ways to treat someone whose blood is excessively thin from Coumadin. From the most conservative which is to watch and wait, and just hold a couple of doses, to the most aggressive way, which is fresh frozen plasma. The intermediate way is Vitamin K.

A therapeutic INR is typically between 2 and 3 with patients with atrial fibrillation (people with artificial heart valves have a standard INR between 2.5 and 3.5, running a bit higher than most others). Let's look at some examples. A patient comes in with an INR of 5, or the patient goes to their physician and they do routine monitoring of their INR, and it comes back at 5, but the patient has no complaints. Typically under that scenario, the patient would hold the Coumadin for a day or two and have it rechecked. If the patient was taking 5 mg of Coumadin per day, it would be reasonable to lower that to 3 or 4 mg per day, then recheck in a few days. If the same patient came in with an INR of 5 or 6 and noticed some blood in her urine, you would check the urine. The report shows it has too numerous to count red blood cells. A more aggressive approach of giving vitamin

K would then be taken. Vitamin K is a direct antagonist to Coumadin and can be given orally, intramuscularly, or intravenously. The dosing regimen ranges anywhere from 1 mg to 10 mg. Vitamin K is a slow reverser of elevated INRs. It normally takes hours to make the INR go down. People are a bit hesitant about covering someone with Vitamin K because even though it may take a couple of hours to get the INR down, it really takes days for that fat soluble vitamin to be cleared from the system. So, it may help lower the INR, but would be tricky to get them therapeutic.

Fresh frozen plasma gives the patient the clotting factors that have been deactivated by the Coumadin. It works rapidly to get the patient's INR down. There are recommendations on the best way to lower someone's INR if it is high. Some pretty consistent recommendations have to do with the patient's INR being elevated but do not have bleeding. In that case we would be more conservative by holding the dose or possibly giving a very low dose of oral Vitamin K. If they are bleeding, you really need to use Vitamin K and fresh frozen plasma. If a patient falls and hits their head while on Coumadin, we had to reverse an intracranial hemorrhage. Most recently, I had someone who came in with bleeding into the right eye because their INR became so high. I typically defer judgment on how to reverse anticoagulation to the specialists, yet it is standard that for a patient on Coumadin vitamin K would give a slow reversal, and the fresh frozen plasma would be more of a fast reversal of bleeding.

Of interest are patients who have a hip fracture, have atrial fibrillation or an artificial valve and need surgery. These patients would be admitted to the hospital and typically a specialist would give recommendations on this, but is very common that before going to the operating room, a hit of fresh frozen plasma would reverse them rather quickly. They go to the operating room, have the surgery, and when the come out of the surgery, they will need to be anti-coagulated again. That is where typically they would use heparin in a drip form and oral Coumadin. The Coumadin will take a couple days to become therapeutic, but in the meantime, their blood will be kept therapeutically thin with the heparin.

In emergency medicine, heparin is a way to thin a patient's blood quickly. Patients who classically need to be anticoagulated quickly are those with acute coronary syndrome or deep venous thrombosis or pulmonary embolism. Heparin is a medication that is given as a bolus and then a drip. It is quite common to give the patient a 5,000 unit bolus and then run the drip at 1,000 per hour, but it is more perfect to do it as a weight based medicine and give the patient 80 units per kilogram bolus, and then run the drip at 18 units per kilogram per hour. The advantage of the heparin is that it can be turned off quickly. Therefore, if the patient starts having bleeding complications, you can turn the heparin drip off and their blood returns to normal in about an hour. On the other side of the coin, once you anticoagulate a person with heparin drip, their blood gets thinned out in approximately an hour. Another way to thin out blood is with subcutaneous Lovenox. This medication is given as a 1 mg per kg subcutaneous injection twice per day. Luvenox works a bit more consistently and anti-coagulates a bit better than heparin. The problem with Lovenox is that once it is on board, you cannot reverse it, or it is very difficult to reverse.

Let's talk about blood transfusions. One unit of blood equals approximately 250 cc of packed red blood cells (PRBCs). One unit equals approximately 10% of a patient's blood volume. Some terms to be aware of: Serum is basically the junk left over. It does not contain clotting factors and does not contain formed elements. Plasma contains the clotting factors. Fresh frozen plasma is what we would use to reverse Coumadin problems. Any time we want to give someone a blood transfusion, we would have to discuss the risks with the patient. Fever is the most common and happens in probably about 25% of the patients who get a blood transfusion. It is more of an allergic-like phenomenon and we can treat them with Benadryl or Tylenol. All patients are concerned with blood-born diseases such as Hepatitis B, C or HIV. I would give the patients the advice that our blood is very well screened now, much better than it used to be. The chance of getting HIV through blood transfusions is approximately 2 in a million. The last thing I would warn the patient about is a catastrophic hemolytic reaction which would occur if we accidentally gave them the wrong blood. But, I always remind the patients that the benefits far outweigh the risks.

The doses we have been talking about above for heparin and Lovenox are anticoagulation doses. There are also deep venous thrombosis prophylaxis doses. These are people who are in bed for a prolonged period of time, and we want to use a mild blood thinner to prevent them from having blood clots in their legs or lungs. A standardized dose for heparin is 5,000 units subcutaneous twice per day or Lovenox 30 mg subcutaneous twice per day. So, once again, those are very low doses compared to anticoagulation doses, but has been shown to reduce the risk of forming a venous thrombosis and potentially a life-threatening complication of pulmonary embolism.

CHAPTER 8

DIABETES

"HONEY, AWHHHH SUGAR, SUGAR"

There are four basic players that clinically are important to us when dealing with of glycemic control. The pancreas secretes insulin and drops glucose and glucagon (a hormone that increases blood glucose). The liver converts glycogen to glucose (also known as gluconeogenesis) and raises blood glucose. The gastrointestinal tract absorbs carbohydrates, thus increasing blood glucose and cortisol from the adrenal gland which is a steroid that increases blood glucose.

Hypoglycemia presents with altered mental status, confusion and anxiety. These patients can have focal neurologic deficits, and this may mimic a cerebrovascular incident or stroke. Most often it occurs when a diabetic has too much insulin or too much of their oral diabetic medications and/or a reduced intake of calories. In any diabetic who is going through an extreme stress response, such as a stroke or a myocardial infarction, the stress response can cause a patient to be hypoglycemic. Just recently in the emergency room, I had a lady who had become hypoglycemic at home. She was confused and had altered mental status, which is why she presented to the emergency department. When we evaluated her, we really could not find a reason as to why her blood sugars dropped. After working her up we did find her troponin to be high and she had a myocardial infarction but no chest pain. When I was working as a house officer, it would not be uncommon to get the phone call from a nurse asking to have some Ativan or a benzodiazepine because a patient had become agitated. What is really important here is to realize that patients who are hypoxic or are hypoglycemic will have anxiety or be agitated. So, a very classic response is to check a blood sugar and check anoxygen saturation and call back. If both are normal, then we can give her a little bit of Xanax. A patient who is hypoglycemic or who is hypoxic can become squirrely and a nurse who is not picking up on this can call and get benzodiazepine ordered. Benzodiazepine causes the patient to become quite sick. So, be careful about thinking a patient just has anxiety when they could have some kind of systemic organic problem.

Patients who are hypoglycemic are treated with calories, either orally, sublingually or through an IV. Typically, if they are asymptomatic or have very minimal symptoms, we will give them oral replacement such as a glass of orange juice with some sugar in it and give them a solid meal like a sandwich. If someone is symptomatic, we would give one amp of dextrose which is about 25 g of glucose. As an FYI, 1 amp of dextrose equals approximately 25 g of glucose, and that equals approximately 200 calories. One glass of orange juice has about 170 calories in it, which is a slower release. So, here is the issue. We have a patient who is hypoglycemic, we give an IV shot of dextrose. What that is going to do is increase blood sugars rapidly to a sharp spike but in some degree of response, even with diabetics, there will be a counter hormonal response to rapidly drop that sugar. It is not uncommon to have someone hypoglycemic, and when we give them a shot of IV dextrose, it rapidly raises their sugar then rapidly drops their sugar, so two hours later they are hypoglycemic again. A better approach would be to give them some orange juice with sugar in it and a couple of crackers, which would create a slower release and not prompt rapid rebound hypoglycemia.

Hypoglycemia falls into multiple categories, including glucose intolerance, gestational diabetes, insulin-dependent diabetes, Type 1 or non insulin-dependent diabetes Type 2. Glucose intolerance is means the body is sluggish to respond to hypoglycemia, but we are not really quite considering them diabetic. These people would be considered pre-diabetics. Gestational diabetics is diabetes strictly related to pregnancy. Women are tested for this and have a problem with having excessively large babies. What happens is that there are so many calories in their body that the baby gets so many calories because of sugar floating around, they become disproportionately large. Lots of times they end up being delivered by C-section. Non insulin-dependent diabetes is where there is not enough insulin from the pancreas or the insulin receptors, and the muscles are not functioning well enough. There are multiple tests to determine whether someone is non-insulin diabetic, including a fasting blood glucose of greater than 1 to 20, random blood glucose greater than 140, or a glycosylated hemoglobin that is elevated. It is said that symptomatic patients who come in with blood glucose of greater than 200, that is diagnostic.

Hyperglycemia has to do with three polys: polydipsia, polyphagia, and polyuria. These are people who really cannot eat or drink enough. They drink incessantly and urinate a lot. Those are symptoms of hyperglycemia. Working in the emergency room, I can tell you that patients who have blurred vision or visual symptoms could be presenting signs of someone who is a diabetic as well as some of the catastrophic problems with diabetes.

About four months ago I had a patient in his late 40s who complained of feeling weak. When he came in by ambulance, he looked entirely too good to be bothering the ambulance crew because he looked so good. He said he had been weak for three days. When I evaluated him, I asked what he meant by being weak for three days and he said he was not able to get off the couch. I had the feeling that this gentleman was malingering, saying he could not get off the couch because he was too weak. I thought I would trick him by asking how he went to the bathroom. He said he had to urinate into a cup.

Now, he had my attention. I asked him again what he meant by saying he was weak. He said he could not take a step without having shortness of breath. At this point, he really had my attention. We started a cardiac work up and, by protocol, the first thing that was done was an EKG. This was put in front of me, and it became clear that this gentleman had a subacute inferior wall myocardial infarction. This gentleman had no history of any past medical problems, and when I got a good story from him, a focus story about chest pain or pressure or anything that may have had him present with presenting signs of acute myocardial infarction, he said no. I immediately had the nurse check a fingerstick on him, and his blood sugar was 300. He went on to explain that he has not seen a doctor in about 10 years. So, this gentleman had undiagnosed diabetes and had a silent myocardial infarction from that.

I once had an 8-year-old who presented with vomiting. He looked like a severe gastroenteritis, but when we worked him up, he was indeed an insulin dependent diabetic and in diabetic ketoacidosis. So, remember that with diabetics, all bets are off with a lot of the presenting problems such as myocardial infarction or peritonitis in the belly. They can have no symptoms or atypical symptoms in the chest and very little physical findings in the abdomen.

In order to understand diabetic medications, you really have to understand the four players in diabetes: the liver, the pancreas, the muscles or receptors in the muscles, and finally, the gastrointestinal tract. We really want to use one medicine from each category and if we are going to use two different medications, we want to attack two different sites. So, again the liver blocks gluconeogenesis, and the medication that does that is Glucophage. This is in the class of the biguanides. The pancreas secretes insulin, so there we want a sulfonylureas or Prandin. Basically, this is just like giving them insulin. You want to take the receptors on the muscles which make them work better. These are the glitazones (TZD). Lastly, is the gastrointestinal tract. So, we can use a medication that blocks carbohydrate absorption such as Precose.

There is overwhelming support for intensive therapy in diabetes. I say this very humbly because my paradigm of medicine is emergency critical care. I do not do outpatient. I did have a lecturer suggest this one time, and I feel pretty strongly that this is the right way to go. A patient presents to the office and you diagnose them with diabetes. Blood sugars are 200. The normal typical medical approach is to tell them to go home, eat better and exercise, and you are putting it in the patient's brain that if you go home and are a good, compliant patient, you might be able to fix this on your own. The reality is that an almost insignificant number can really do this. What happens is that a couple months later, the patient comes back with high blood sugars, weight gain, and worse overall cholesterol, it then becomes kind of a parental issue for me when I say the patient did not do what I suggested. Then the patient feels like they are punished when placed on medication.

There is literature that shows obese women have a higher incidence of ovarian cancer, and the thought was that it was the estrogen secreted from the fatty cells of being obese that contributed to this higher rate of cancer. Apparently, when this was looked at in more detail, it turned out not to be that the adipose tissue was secreting more estrogen. Actually, obese women were less likely to get regular follow ups at their gynecologist's office, and the reason quoted was they felt the negative feelings from their provider of having to do a pelvic exam on someone who is obese. Thus, they did not seek care as much as non-obese women. This point was used to demonstrate why intensive therapy in diabetics is such a good thing. If you are going to care for a diabetic on a regular basis, you really want to create a strong therapeutic relationship with them. If a patient comes in who is mildly obese, with high blood sugars, you know they are diabetic. If you started them on Glucophage right away instead of giving them the one-month or two-month grace period to go home and try it themselves, they could fail 99 out of 100 times. Instead, put them on a glucose medication such as Glucophage, say "go home, diet, exercise, and start taking this medication," when they come back in a month, they are going to look better. They are going to have lost weight because of the Glucophage, which has a tendency to make them lose weight. You are going to be freaked out and excited with what a good job they have done. They might have to do more, but they did such a good job it is very exciting. Therefore, you have engaged, energetic patients rather than ones who feel chastised. It is not uncommon to have patients lie about their blood sugars. They come possibly even making up false numbers to satisfy their provider.

It is important to talk about metabolic syndrome, also known as Syndrome X, which is a metabolic complication of high insulin states. Metabolic syndrome has to do with high insulin states, obesity and hyperlipidemia. These all seem to go together. Someone with too much insulin or excessive insulinwill gain weight, and their cholesterol will get crazy. If we give them insulin injections, they will gain weight, cholesterol will go bad, and there is not really much they can do about it. It is just how Mother Nature made our bodies work. On the opposite side of the coin, that is how the Adkins diet works. People who have very low carbohydrates get very low insulin levels and therefore they lose weight rapidly. You can expect any patient starting on an insulin regimen to gain weight. Also, if you put a patient on a medication that attacks the pancreas such as sulfonylureas or Prandin, it is similar to giving them insulin where they will have the metabolic syndrome as well.

Type 2 diabetics who take pills are prone to being a "HONKers." This is hyperosmolar nonketotic coma. These patients present extremely hyperglycemic but not in an acidotic state. Therefore, they would have no anion gap. These patients need aggressive IV fluids and small amounts of insulin. So, if a patient came in and was in a hyperosmolar nonketotic state with a blood sugar of 650, and once again not acidotic, these patients need 5, 6, 7 liters of fluid and just about 4-6 units of IV insulin. The primary problem is that they are dehydrated, not that they are suffering from a deficiency of insulin cell. Give aggressive IV fluids, place a Foley in and monitor ins and outs. Remember, the limiting factor for IV fluids is congestive heart failure. So, you just want to keep a close eye on oxygen saturations.

Insulin dependent diabetics (juvenile onset diabetes) really have no pancreatic function and are insulin dependent. The pancreas normally secretes about 25-50 units per day of insulin. Regular insulin is the only insulin that can be given IV. The onset of regular insulin is about 30 minutes to an hour and normally spikes in about 2-4 hours. 70/30 insulin means 70% of the insulin is medium acting where 30% of the insulin is short acting. Medium onset insulin has onset of approximately 1-4 hours and spikes in 6-10 hours. So, if a patient had 10 units of 70/30 insulin, about 7 units is medium acting and 3 units is short acting. Therefore, it should cover the patient for approximately 12 hours. It is the insulin dependent diabetics who present with diabetic ketoacidosis where the mnemonic for how to care for them is **VEGA**. V stands for volume or they need IV fluids. E stands for electrolytes which is potassium. G is glucose where we would treat with an insulin drip. A is the acidosis which basically means we do not stop the insulin drip until their acidosis resolves.

V	**VOLUME**
E	**ELECTROLYTES (POTASSIUM)**
G	**GLUCOSE (INSULIN)**
A	**ACIDOSIS**

Treating patients with diabetic ketoacidosis would require

a 24 hour lecture in and of itself. They take intensive monitoring just because you have to watch their blood sugars and electrolytes so closely. These patients come in needing massive onset of IV fluids but also need an insulin drip. Now, it is very common for people in metabolic acidosis to have hyperkalemia, and as we are treating these patients with the insulin drip, and their blood sugar starts to slowly go down, so will their potassium. So, patients who are being monitored in diabetic ketoacidosis, as their blood sugar comes down, their potassium will drop, and we know that the potassium is just going to get worse, so when a potassium normalizes, in the IV fluids we will start adding potassium just to make sure that they do not become hypokalemic.

CHAPTER 9

IV FLUIDS AND OTHER ELECTROLYTE STUFF

There are three main body compartments where fluid resides. We first have the extracellular fluid, in the vasculature and the interstitium. The interstitium is the area between the cells, also known as our third space. Then, we have our intracellular fluid, which is the fluid within our cells. So, there are two main categories of extracellular fluid and intracellular fluid. In the extracellular fluid, we have two different spots, the vascular bed and the interstitium. Fluid is constantly circulating between compartments trying to find homeostasis. Know that fat really is negligible intracellular fluid. If someone is massively obese, it does not mean that they have a higher volume of water in their body than a non-obese person.

The main hormones that are responsible for fluid balance are antidiuretic hormone and aldosterone. An antidiuretic hormone, also known as vasopressin, at higher doses is really stimulated by the osmolality of the concentration of all solute particles in a solution. When antidiuretic hormone is going crazy, it is going to have us retain water and not pee it out. Think about the concept of the name: antidiuretic hormone. If we give a patient a diuretic, of course they would pee. If we gave them an antidiuretic, they would not pee. Something interesting about antidiuretic hormone is that if you have a patient who is stabbed in the spleen and is bleeding out internally, their sympathetic nervous system would go crazy where epinephrine would give a staying alive response. Antidiuretic hormone would kick in as well. At low doses, as the bleeding starts, anti-diuretic hormone would start getting secreted and cause us not to pee. As the antidiuretic hormone comes out in higher concentrations, we now call it vasopressin, which means it causes our blood vessels to vasoconstrict as well as retaining our volume. So, it is a hormone that does help preserve life. Aldosterone, which is secreted by the adrenal glands, is stimulated by blood volume and blood sodium. When aldosterone is working overtime, it causes us to retain sodium or reabsorb sodium in the kidneys, thus kicking out potassium. As a side note, we do use a medicine called Aldactone or spironolactone, which actually blocks aldosterone. We call this a potassium sparing diuretic so it does the opposite of aldosterone. It causes sodium to leave the body and thus water will follow it while retaining potassium. Aldactone is a medication we use in relatively severe cases of congestive heart failure. With these people, you can have a problem with hyperkalemia, again because spironolactone is a potassium-sparing diuretic causing potassium to be elevated.

In discussing the relationship between food compartments, hydrostatic pressure and oncotic pressure are two that we need to know. The hydrostatic pressure is basically just the pressure in the pump. The pressure in the vascularity that causes fluid to go forward and backward. The second pressure is your oncotic pressure, which is controlled by serum protein or albumin. If a patient has a lower albumin state, you can give them fluids left and right, but the fluid is going to weep out into their interstitium at the expense of the vascular bed. Someone who is malnourished or in liver failure and has a very low albumin state and cannot produce the albumin in the liver; they can be euvolemic yet be dehydrated because all of the volume is in their interstitium and is not staying in their blood vessels. Therefore, if you have someone who comes in with massively swollen legs, it is by far most common that they are in congestive heart failure or have some degree of right heart failure. They could also have low albumin states. With these people, you can give them volume all you want to, but unless you replace some degree of serum osmolality (albumin), they will not be able to pull that volume back into their blood vessels.

In discussing osmolality, the normal range of osmolality is 280 to 300 millimoles per kilogram. As you will recall, the first step in working up a patient who is hyponatremic is to check serum osmolality and make sure it is not a false osmole in the blood that is causing the sodium to be abnormally low. Osmolality is calculated. It has to do with three main components of blood which is our sodium, our glucose and our urea. It is from serum osmolality and calculating an osmolality gap that we would identify patients who are overdosed with heavy alcohol such as ethylene, glycyl methanol, isopropyl alcohol. These patients would present with some kind of toxic congestion and in working them up, you would find their serum osmolality that we calculate by a formula to be grossly different than the lab's calculation of serum osmolality. It is from there that we would go into heavy alcohol work up.

Here's the nitty-gritty on IV fluid's. There are two types of IV fluids, known as crystalloids and colloids. Crystalloids contain electrolytes or crystals. Colloids contain plasma proteins. For the rest of your career, you will pretty much only use crystalloids. (Colloids involve giving proteins like albumin or synthetic protein and is done in the intensive care unit.) Isotonic means the same osmolality as blood such as normal saline or lactated ringers. Normal saline has 0.9% of sodium chloride. Lactated ringers have more electrolytes and glucose in it. Note that surgeons love lactated ringers based on their training. If you have a patient with abdominal pain and you think they are going to go into the operating room, it is wise just to change them right over to lactated ringers, instead of normal saline. As an FYI about normal saline, you can give ½ normal saline or ¼ normal saline if you are concerned about giving less sodium. The only time we would be concerned about this is with a patient who has congestive heart failure.

When talking about when to give someone IV fluids, there are all these fancy formulas that residents need to learn while they are in school, but as soon as they get out they realize those formulas are not as applicable to care as they first thought. IV fluid really is an art. It is difficult to tell how much IV fluid a patient truly needs without invasive monitoring. We need to know the three things we can give IV, and we need to calculate those needs for every patient. We can give them fluid or water. We can give them electrolytes. Or, we can give them calories, which is glucose. Now, if the patient is dehydrated, we would give them fluids. Fluid comes in any of our IV solutions. So, if you give them normal saline, you are giving them quite a bit of free fluid. The electrolytes have to do with sodium and chloride, we can always add potassium to our IV fluids. Calories we can give dextrose solution or D5 normal saline, which is dextrose with normal saline.

The real limit on fluids is congestive heart failure. If we give them too much fluid, it puts them into congestive heart failure. It never looks good in the emergency room when, after aggressively hydrating a patient, they are become short of breath and wheezy, and we have to take some of the fluid back with Lasix.

CHAPTER 10

ARTERIAL BLOOD GAS AND
OTHER RESPIRATORY STUFF

The first test before doing a blood gas is called an Allen test. To do this, grab the patient's wrist and occlude the radial and ulnar arteries to actually cut off circulation in the hand. The arterial blood gas is done in the radial artery, and this test checks the patency of the artery. So, what we would do is pinch off the radial and ulnar artery and then let go of the ulnar artery to see if the ulnar artery adequately perfuses the hand. The concept here is that if we do an arterial blood gas and cause damage to the radial artery such as an aneurysm or thrombus, the ulnar artery will still be able to perfuse the hand and would not become necrotic. The Allen test should be done before every blood gas even though clinically I rarely seen it done. The concept is to make sure the hand has good blood flow from the radial and ulnar artery. When we ventilate the blood gas, there are three main values that are important to us to make clinical decisions. Only three. We want the pH, which shows whether the patient is acidic or alkalotic (normal range is approximately 7.35-7.45) we want the PC02 and we want the P02. When we get this a little more exact, we are really concerned here with one value, the PC02. So, it is my contention that the most important value we can get from a blood gas is the patient's carbon dioxide level.

PC02 or carbon dioxide will tell us if a patient is retaining or blowing off carbon dioxide. As an FYI, if pH and PC02 go in the opposite direction, the acid base disorder is respiratory. For example, if the pH is low and the carbon dioxide is high, it is a respiratory acidosis. On the opposite side of the coin, if the arrows are going in the same direction, it is a metabolic problem. If the pH is low and the PC02 is low, that is more of a metabolic acidosis. In discussing the terminology of acid base, remember that oxygenation has to do with the exchange of oxygen where ventilation has to do with the exchange of carbon dioxide. It is important that you understand carbon dioxide is an acid, and under the worst case scenarios, carbon dioxide will rise in the body approximately 3 mm of mercury per minute. Therefore, if we have a patient who has chronic obstructive pulmonary disease and on hypoxic drive, and we give them oxygen at high levels, it will cause them to hypo-ventilate and thus retain carbon dioxide. It is the hypoxic patient with chronic obstructive pulmonary disease who must be observed closely. If a patient with chronic obstructive pulmonary disease who retains carbon dioxide is given high-flow oxygen to keep their oxygen levels up, they can slowly become obtunded, sleepy and poorly aroused; the only way to really fix them is with positive pressure ventilation such as BIPAP or intubation.

Carbon dioxide will rise for two main reasons: the first is hypoventilation from chronic obstructive pulmonary disease or narcotics, and the second is an obstruction such as pneumonia or congestive heart failure. Know that there are two ways to decrease carbon dioxide in patients with severe respiratory failure. We need to remove the obstruction so we can use Lasix or antibiotics or Proventil or positive pressure ventilation such as CPAP or intubation. BIPAP means biphasic positive airway pressure. CPAP means continuous positive airway pressure. What we need to know here is BIPAP is used to oxygenate a patient and ventilate them to help with oxygen exchange and carbon dioxide exchange. CPAP is used more to oxygenate. The only time I have ever seen this used is with sleep apnea patients at night.

There is a concept called pickwickian syndrome. These people have so much body fat that it makes it actually difficult to breathe. This syndrome is named after a character in Charles Dickens' book, *The Pickwick Papers*. Mr. Pickwick was a man who was so obese that he wheezed and gasped while breathing. In discussing P02 or oxygenation, P02 is normally greater than 80 mm of mercury. The best way to tell if someone is not oxygenating well is by checking 02 saturation. It should be considered your fifth vital sign, and done for any patient with any kind of pulmonary symptoms. 02 saturation is measured with a clothes- pin like clamp that fits on the patient's finger. You put it on, and it measures a patient's oxygen level. There is a very close correlation between oxygen saturation and P02. You can get false elevations of 02 saturation in patients with carbon monoxide poisoning or methemoglobinemia. You can also get false lows with oxygen saturation with fingernail polish, low flow states to the patient's arms like in someone with Raynaud's syndrome or someone who is excessively cold. I have been fooled a couple of times to be watching a patient whom I feel is critically ill and all of a sudden see their oxygen saturation start dropping just to realize they have a blood pressure cuff on that arm that was automatically inflating to check the blood pressure, thus cutting off blood flow to that finger.

So, out of all three of the measurements, it is my contention that the most important number is the carbon dioxide. We can gage pH from a venous pH. If you really want to know the patient's acid base status, you can do a venous blood gas where the venous pH and the arterial pH are almost exactly the same. Remember that carbon dioxide is an acid and in venous blood, you have more carbon dioxide in it than the arterial blood, and the difference is about 0.02 from how acidic a venous sample will be relative to an arterial sample. So, if I really need to know someone's pH and could get a venous pH done, that would tell me where the acid base status is. Oxygenation I can get from an 02 saturation. But, again, the only way I can really get a vitally important carbon dioxide level is to do an arterial blood gas.

How do we increase oxygenation in a patient? How can we fix a patient who comes in hypoxic? We have a number of ways. The first is to give higher flow oxygen. Normal room oxygen, normal atmospheric oxygen, is approximately 21%. We can always give them more oxygen either through nasal cannula or a non-rebreather mask. Next, we can fix an oxygenation problem with bronchodilators such as Albuterol or Proventil which stimulates beta-2 receptor, or we can give them ipratropium or Atrovent which is an anti-cholinergic, which relaxes the bronchials through a nebulizer treatment. We can do this typically with pneumonia, chronic obstructive pulmonary disease, or asthma, as well as heart failure. We can increase oxygen is by taking away some of the obstruction with diuretics such as Lasix. We can also redistribute the fluid that is in their lungs by giving them nitroglycerin. In the most extreme states, we can intubate them. Note that there is very good evidence for the BIPAP, especially with congestive heart failure patients. So, using BIPAP early may save a patient having intubation.

CHAPTER 11

CEREBRAL SPINAL FLUID
(LUMBAR PUNCTURE)

Why would we do a lumbar puncture? There are really three main symptoms we would look for; two in the emergency room. We want to look for a bleed or subarachnoid hemorrhage, or we are looking for meningitis (infection). The last reason for lumbar puncture is to find inflammatory problems and autoimmune disease such as multiple sclerosis. Of interest is a spinal headache. These are patients who recently had some kind of lumbar puncture done, and when the needle was put through the meninges, the hole did not quite close and now the patient has cerebral spinal fluid that leaks out. These patients have debilitating headaches when they stand up. When they lie down, the pain is almost resolved. But, when they stand up, they are in debilitating pain. Of absolute fascination to me is how this is fixed. An anesthesiologist will do a venepuncture in the patient's arm and take out about 10-20 cc of blood. They will find the site that the lumbar puncture was done and inject the blood right there at the site. Now, the blood will surround that hole in the meninges and stop the leaking of fluid. This must be a pressure gradient that is immediately changed because these patients almost immediately feel better. It is like night and day, how they go from being debilitatingly sick to feeling better. It is quite an amazing concept.

When we talk about bleeding or subarachnoid hemorrhage, we will do a lumbar puncture actually looking for blood in the sample. There are two reasons why you would have blood in the cerebral spinal fluid. One is a traumatic tap and the other is because there is indeed a subarachnoid hemorrhage. Now, when we do a lumbar puncture, we are actually going to fill up four different tubes of cerebral spinal fluid, labeled 1-4. If you have someone who has 10-20 red blood cells in the first sample but no red blood cells in the last sample, you can safely assume that the blood in the first tube was from a traumatic tap. If you have 10-20 red blood cells and all four of the tubes, under the right clinical setting, that suggests subarachnoid hemorrhage. When looking at subarachnoid hemorrhage, note that a CAT scan is approximately 95% diagnostic. So, if a patient comes in with the classic symptoms of a thunder clap-like headache, acute onset of headache that is the worst headache of their life, especially if they have a rigid neck, these patients need a CAT scan initially. If the CAT scan shows subarachnoid hemorrhage, then your job is done, and the patient needs to be sent to a neurosurgeon.

If the CAT scan is negative, but they clinically have the appearance of a subarachnoid hemorrhage, they need a lumbar puncture. With a lumbar puncture, we are looking for one of two things: either blood (as we talked about before) in a spun-down specimen, or what is called a xanthochromia. Xanthochromia is a yellowish pigment that is found after red blood cell analysis. So, if you have multiple red blood cells in the cerebral spinal fluid and they start breaking down, it will release a yellowish pigment, which can be picked up by a lab technician who looks at the sample. Any patient for the rest of your career who presents with a headache is indeed a subarachnoid hemorrhage until proven otherwise. So, any patient who presents with a headache that occurred in a high-stress environment, and I do not mean emotionally stressful, but physically stressful such as lifting weights, lifting or moving something heavy, orduring intercourse when there is high intracerebral pressure, if they come in with a headache and the story was that it occurred while there was pressure being put on their cerebral vessels, you need to take them very seriously for subarachnoid hemorrhage.

When working up a patient with infection or infectious meningitis, and we do a lumbar puncture, we are looking for white blood cells, neutrophils, protein and glucose in the cerebral spinal fluid. If there is a bacterial infection, they are going to have a lot of white blood cells and a large number of neutrophils. Bacterial infections have a tendency to want to gobble up the glucose, so the glucose will be low and protein will be high. When we do cerebral spinal fluid for inflammatory or autoimmune problems, we are really looking for oligoclonal gamma globulins, which helps diagnose multiple sclerosis.

Contraindications for lumbar puncture are increased intracranial pressure, as seen in someone with a brain tumor, severe degenerative joint disease where you would have a very difficult time getting the spinal fluid needed through the disc space, or a bad site which means they have an infection on their back, and by doing a lumbar puncture, you could actually take the infection from the skin and move it into the cerebrospinal space.

When doing a lumbar puncture, you want to record opening pressures. Someone with a high pressure in the cerebral spinal fluid can suggest certain pathologies as opposed to others. The four tubes that we use have to do with chemistries, culture and sensitivity, microscopic evaluation and the last one is reserved for special studies such as antigen studies.

CHAPTER 12

DEMYSTIFYING THE CHEST AND ABDOMINAL RADIOGRAPH

In reviewing this next material, I would like you to forget any preconceptions that you have about chest radiographs. I would recommend that you use the following information and the system that is used to interpret a chest radiograph to increase your confidence.

Let's talk about John's first rule. This rule is to *really look* at a radiograph. It should take two minutes to evaluate a chest radiograph. I like thinking of it as going to a comedy show where it is free to get in, but there is a two-drink minimum. Any time you order a chest radiograph, you need to devote two minutes to thoroughly review the radiograph. I have found many times in my career where I did indeed miss something, whether it was an infiltrate or a pneumothorax or fractured ribs. It was not that I could not see, it was because I did not take my time and was going too fast. So, I have to stress that if you are going to be a speedster when it comes to looking at chest radiographs, you are going to miss something. It is not a matter of if you are going to miss something, it is a matter of when and how big of a miss is it going to be. So, I cannot stress enough to take your time and take the two-minute rule. So, if you order five chest radiographs in a day, 10 minutes out of your shift should be specifically directed toward reading radiographs.

The second philosophical point I would tell you about when interpreting a chest radiograph is that the eyes see what the mind knows. That is a theme we are going to come back to when discussing diagnostic imagery. The eyes see what the mind knows, meaning that the mind may perceive a patient a very particular way, and you are going to look at the radiograph based on Bayes theorem or pretest probability (after looking at the patient, how do we expect the chest radiograph to look?) If a patient presents clinically in congestive heart failure with a history of congestive heart failure, is on 80 mg twice per day of Lasix, ACE inhibitor and Coreg, has jugular venous distention and pedal edema, so everything clinically about this patient says they are in congestive heart failure. Let's take it a step further. We give them nitroglycerin and Lasix, and it completely makes them better. So, clinically, we are absolute sure that this patient is in congestive heart failure. When the technician brings the film to us to evaluate after we saw the patient, it may skew how we look at the film. When the patient is clinically in congestive heart failure, we should have a very good idea of what the chest radiograph is going to look like, and we are just using the film to confirm it and to rule out other problems.

The same could be said of someone who comes in with arm pain. Now, if this is someone who got struck with a bat or fell off a bicycle and has a gross deformity to the forearm, it is easy. You are just looking at the x-ray to confirm that they do indeed have a fracture. Let's say it is someone who started working a new job and has a lot of twisting motions. There was no acute trauma, but they come in with arm pain. The pretest probability that there is a fracture is going to be extremely low and therefore would count that pretest probability in when reviewing the chest radiograph. So, once again, the eyes see what the mind knows. Clinically, you should know why you are doing a study and have a good idea of what you are going to see before you look at the film.

You need a system, not just with the radiographs but also with the EKGs. You need a very consistent systematic approach so you will not miss anything. I would like to offer you John's **ROAR RIP'T ABC's** approach. Again, I would suggest you apply this with every radiograph that you interpret for the rest of your career as well as the two-minute rule. So, if you apply this system and take two minutes out of your day to do this with every chest radiograph, you will become more confident and more proficient at dealing with chest films. We are going to discuss **ROAR**. This is the easy one. **ROAR** stands for right patient, old x-rays, alignment and right date.

R	**RIGHT PATIENT**
O	**OLD X-RAYS**
A	**ALIGNMENT**
R	**RIGHT DATE**

This is where you are going to spend just a 10-20 seconds validating the data, making sure that you do indeed have the right patient, are there old x-rays to compare it with, if the film is hung correctly, and that you have the right date. Now, for the past few years I have been working at smaller hospitals and when I order an x-ray it may be the only one that x-ray has done in the last 10-15 minutes. At a bigger hospital, you do an x-ray, go down to look at it, and only one film is hanging. If you are assuming this is your patient's film, you are going to get burned sooner or later. So, take the time to ensure that you have the right date and the right patient. If there are old films to compare with, you want them handy so if there are any abnormalities, you can compare and contrast them. Here is a pearl for you. If you are evaluating a radiograph, and in the review of the old films, you see multiple different films of multiple different body systems and there is not a good explanation, (the patient is a stunt bike rider) it implies to me the patient derives secondary gain from the medical system (in other words, they are crazy.)

Then we come to the beef of our interpretation of the film. Now, the **RIP'T** stands for evaluation of the quality of the radiograph. R is rotation. I is inspiration. P is penetration. T is technique.

R	ROTATION
I	INSPIRATION
P	PENETRATION
T	TECHNIQUE

Let's talk about that in more detail. With rotation, we want to see if the clavicles line up, like the sight on a gun, behind the spinous process. There should be equal distance between the spinous process and the end of the clavicle, the medial aspect of the clavicle. If a patient is twisted and their right shoulder is closer to the x-ray beams and further away from the film than the left shoulder, there will be distortion in anatomy. I am not saying you disqualify a film if it is moderately rotated, but you just need to put that in your data bank or the filter, if you will, for when you review the film. A demented person with very severe kyphosis is not going to be rotated to some degree and you just have to weigh that in when reviewing the films. Inspiration is where we actually count the ribs to make sure we see between 9 and 11 ribs. The deeper a breath they take, the more of the lungs you will be able to see. If a patient is demented and cannot follow instructions to take a deep breath, you will maybe only see six ribs. You will have to weigh in your thought process that they may have pathology lying in the posteroinferior aspects of the lungs that we would not be able to see on a PA radiograph, and a lateral x-ray would be much more helpful.

P is penetration where we want to see the vertebral bodies behind the heart. If the heart is so white or under-penetrated that we cannot see the vertebral bodies, we call this film under-penetrated and is going to be more difficult to interpret the radiograph as opposed to a film that is over-penetrated which means the film is excessively black. Those films are easier to read. When working as a house officer, five years in, I really thought I was becoming good at what I did. I had a consistent problem of not telling if the radiograph was under-penetrated versus congestive heart failure. So, I turned to my senior colleagues, people who were house officer PAs for 20 years, and asked that question. "How can you tell if it is really congestive heart failure versus under-penetrated?" I was really expecting these great words of wisdom to help me differentiate between them. Both of them looked at me and said, "You know, John, I had a tough time with that too." So, with that said, an under-penetrated film can fool you into thinking it is congestive heart failure. But, you really need to weigh in whether you can see the vertebral bodies or not and use pretest probability. How does the patient look?

T is for technique, which is a PA film versus an AP film. PA means posterior-anterior, and AP means anterior-posterior. To explain this concept of posterior and anterior versus anterior and posterior, think of holding your hand up to a flashlight beam that is shining against a white wall. The flashlight beams are the x-ray beams, and the wall is the film. Your hand shadow is going to be what appears on the radiograph. Now, if you take your hand and put it very close to the wall, your shadow is going to be quite crisp and the shadow is going to be almost the exact size of your hand. If you take your hand and move it back towards the flashlight, the shadow will become bigger and will become blurred. It is that same concept that has to do with interpreting a posterior-anterior film versus an anterior-posterior film. Now, the heart lies anterior in the chest, so if you are doing and AP film which means the beam of the x-ray is going from the anterior to the posterior. Take a portable chest x-ray, the heart is lying further away from the film, (which is behind the patient's back) and therefore the heart will be disproportionately big and a bit hazy. A posterior-anterior film is when the patient actually turns their back, puts their back up to the film, and the x-ray beams go posterior-anterior. That is a more perfect film, and you get a better view of the heart, a crisper heart shadow, and therefore a PA film is a much better film than the AP film. So, once again when you are first walking up to a film, you are going to give it two minutes and are going to apply rip-T ror-ing ABCS where rip-T is rotation, inspiration, penetration and technique.

ABC'S is the systematic approach to where your eyes travel on the x-ray. A is air spaces. B is bones and borders. C is cardiovascular and mediastinum. S is soft tissues.

A	**AIR**
B	**BONES & BORDERS**
C	**CARDIOVASCULAR & MEDIASTINUM**
S	**SOFT TISSUES**

When you first start this systematic approach, let me warn you. If you come up and see a goober, something big right off the get go, like there is a large mass in the right chest wall, or let's say a knife wound to the chest with still an impaled foreign body, you need to ignore the goober. Ignore the thing that is screaming out at you, put your hand over it to cover it up, and review the whole film. Then come back to that. Still, every film gets two minutes. Every film gets the systematic approach. Let's talk about air spaces. There are three things we want to look at. We want to look at the gastric bubble. We want to look for free air. And, we want to look at the lung spaces to determine whether they are disproportionately black or disproportionately white. With gastric air in the left upper quadrant, we are just confirming that there is indeed or there is not air in the stomach. Very rarely does this have high clinical utility. I have seen patients with some kind of gastric outlet problem and had so much gastric distention it impeded the left hemidiaphragm and we needed to put an NG tube in to evacuate the stomach so their breathing got better. It is not uncommon for children who are swallowing a lot of air when crying to have a very distended abdomen, again of low clinical utility.

Free air has to do with air that is between the liver and the diaphragm. What you would see is a very thin line in the right upper quadrant that suggests free air in the belly that is isolating the diaphragm. Now, this is only seen on an upright chest radiograph. Remember that we always have to evaluate the films in terms of gravity. Water goes to the bottom and air goes to the top. Now, if you picture this, picture someone who has a right hemithorax. Say this patient was stabbed in the chest, and the lung is half full of blood. If you have an upright chest x-ray, you are going to see a very well delineated line in the middle of the chest where below it is all white suggesting blood. The black line going up suggests the air. Now, that patient's x-ray would look very different if the patient were supine. So, if the films were coming from anterior to posterior position with the patient supine, all that blood is going to layer out so the whole right lung is going to be white as opposed to the well delineated line of someone who is in the upright position.

Finally, we have to look at the lung spaces. This is where we start on the top by the patient's jaw and go side to side and look at the lungs in terms of, do I see anything that looks abnormal? What we are looking for is any area that is disproportionately black compared to the rest of the film or disproportionately white. Now, evaluating the lung spaces does take practice and takes looking at a lot of films. Some pearls I would give to you are to use pretest probability. So, if you see an area in the right lower base that appears a bit hazy and this patient clinically looks like pneumonia and has crackles at the right base, there is a high threshold of calling that a possible infiltrate. I have had students constantly have problems with the hilar area of the lung, looking at it and trying to call pathology there, and my best advice would be "don't." The hilum has to do with multiple branches of blood vessels and multiple degrees of thickness that come right off into the lungs, and this can look asymmetrical and abnormal from patient to patient. I would recommend having discipline and if you see a hilum that looks a little funny, I would say call it normal and 39-40 times you are going to be right. I have seen some hilar adenopathy in the lymph nodes, but overall, I have never gotten myself into trouble not calling pathology in the hilum.

Next is bones and borders. From here, we are going to look at all of the bones. We are going to start at the right clavicle, go through the clavicle, look at the humerus, the head of the humerus, the glenoid. We are going to look at the acromioclavicular joint. From there, you are going to use your fingers and trace every single rib. Here is where you can unfortunately pick up child abuse in a child who has had multiple rib fractures or fractures in multiple stages of healing. From there you would want to look at the vertebral bodies for compression fractures. Then do the same thing on the left side. This is a bit time consuming, but again, the reason you are reading this chapter is because you do not want to miss anything on a radiograph. It is from looking at these bones that you can also see lytic lesions in bones such as hyperparathyroid tumor or multiple myeloma. So, look at all of the bones when reading an x-ray.

B stands for border. You are going to look at the right heart border, right diaphragm border, left heart, left diaphragm border. This is an appropriate time to talk about silhouette sign. Silhouette sign suggests that if you have two substances of the same density and they are touching each other, the border between them will not be there. Again, using a flashlight analogy and a white wall analogy. If you put your hand up (which really is a water density because our body is mostly water) and you take your other hand and put it up, if you hold them 2-3" apart, you will see two very distinct shadows. If you put your hands together and touch each other, you will really only see one shadow of two hands. There will not be a line between them. It is the same thing with radiographs, and this is really helpful when looking for pneumonia. So once again, silhouette sign means that if you have two opacities of the same density that are touching each other, you will not see a clear line between them. Pneumonia is a water density because you have all these germs, and fluid fills the area, and it actually is a puddle of water in the lung. The heart and the diaphragm are made of muscles, which are mostly water as well, and radiographically they appear the same. So, if you have a pneumonia that is touching the right diaphragm, you will see either a very slurred right diaphragm or will see a bump in the right diaphragm. So, it is from bones and borders that we look at the right heart and the right diaphragm, the left heart and left diaphragm looking for continuity of the diaphragm, and if it is broken, you have a high index of suspicion of a water-based opacification, which is normally a pneumonia.

C is for cardiovascular. We need to look at the heart size and whether the patient has an enlarged cardiac silhouette. We are also going to check the cardiothoracic ratio which means you measure the distance from the right side of the heart to the left side of the heart and use that distance to see if that is greater than half of the chest. Specifically, to take that measurement go to one of the spinous processes right behind the heart and measure from there toward the left lateral wall. If that measurement extends past the chest wall, we would refer to that as an enlarged cardiac silhouette. A pearl here is that this is typically called cardiomegaly, and I would suggest to you that probably it is. But, what happens if the heart is not big but there is a large pericardial effusion, which makes the heart look big? The most appropriate term is enlarged cardiac silhouette, not necessarily cardiomegaly. To really determine which, you would have to do an echocardiogram.

Also, under C for cardiovascular, we would look at the mediastinum. We want to see if the mediastinum is disproportionately wide. There are no specific criteria to say if the mediastinum is wide. Some people use the distance of 8 cm. Some people refer to their pager size, meaning is the mediastinum bigger than the pager carried on the hip. So, it is more of a gestalt to determine whether it is big or not and the clinical context of the patient. Remember that there could be a thoracic aneurysm that is traumatic from a rapid deceleration, which is known as aortic disruption or you can have a thoracic dissecting aneurysm which is typically found in older folks with a long-standing history of hypertension. Lastly, from the systematic review, S is soft tissue where we look at the soft tissues in the neck and the breast tissue. Here we are looking for subcutaneous air, primarily looking for any kind of tumors or foreign bodies that may be in the soft tissues, pretty low yield overall, but we want to be thorough.

If we look at a film that is too white where we see a lesion or both lungs that are disproportionately white, the mnemonic here is **PM ACE**. The lesions that are disproportionately white are what we have to clinically assess. P is pneumonia, M is mass, A is atelectasis, C is CHF, and E is effusion (fluid).

P	**PNEUMONIA**
M	**MASS**
A	**ATELECTASIS**
C	**CHF (CONGESTIVE HEART FAILURE)**
E	**EFFUSION (FLUID)**

In pneumonia, we want to look for clinical features and again to use our pretest probability such as a leukocytosis, to determine if they are they hypoxic. We are going to look for an infiltrate on the chest x-ray. Sometimes young, healthy people come in and say they have been coughing terribly, have a high fever, and are bringing up gooky yellow stuff. In these cases, pneumonia is a relatively easy diagnosis. But in the pediatric or neonatal population, as well as elderly folks, it may present as much more subtle.

Once again, 9 out of 10 times, if someone comes in and you are very concerned about a bacterial infection, think wind and water, meaning pneumonia or urinary tract infection. Radiographically, there are three different presentations of pneumonia. We have bronchial pneumonia, alveolar pneumonia and interstitial pneumonia. All of these pneumonias have to do with anatomically where the pneumonia sat in. Did it sit in the bronchial? Did it sit in at the end of the bronchia in the alveolar area? Or, did it weep out through the alveolar area into the interstitial area? Now, when describing this to audiences, I like to use my hand to demonstrate the location of the pneumonia where my arm is actually the bronchial. If you have an infection that sets in the bronchial area, I would like you to think of them as big, bad bugs. They are the more scary bugs. They are the ones that make the patients look most sick.

Now, if the bronchial gets completely occluded, that can decrease the pressure going to the alveolar area. I like to think of the alveolar area as a big bunch of grapes where as you breathe in, the grapes expand, and as you blow out, the grapes shrink to kind of look like raisins. If someone has a bronchial obstruction, we would not have enough pressure to keep those grapes enlarged, therefore would all collapse and that is another term for pneumonia. What I would suggest in a bronchial pneumonia is that these germs are so big, they are like the size of PEAs and block up the bronchial. These are pseudomonas, E-coli, and anaerobes, which can happen in aspiration pneumonia and here is where we would want to put a big flag up for klebsiella, which is classic with alcoholics and staph. The bronchial pneumonia is more of a hospital-acquired problem which might occur in the elderly lady who came to the hospital for hip surgery. She was doing quite well, but then on day three came up with fever, white count, hypoxia and a big infiltrate. In such cases, we would want to be quite aggressive in treating for pseudomonas.

Now, alveolar pneumonia has to do with an infection down "in the hand" or in "the grapes" area. My mnemonic there is

SHZAM. S is strep pneumo. H is haemophilus influenzae. Z is just to fill in the mnemonic. A stands for a-typicals. M is for Moraxella catarrhalis.

S	**STREP PNEUMO**
H	**HAEMOPHILUS**
Z	**is just for "zee" space**
A	**ATYPICALS**
M	**MORAXELLA**

This is your classic community-acquired pneumonia. This is someone who comes in off the street with fever, cough and whose x-ray shows pneumonia. Any patient who comes in with community-acquired pneumonia needs to be treated for the different classes of germs, including gram positives, gram negatives and atypicals. The most common way to treat them is either with a macrolide antibiotic (non-erythromycin because erythromycin does not cover gram negatives), fluoroquinolone antibiotic (ciprofloxacin does not cover strep pneumo well), or combination therapy of something like a third generation cephalosporin and a macrolide. Now, it is alveolar pneumonia that predisposes patients to air bronchograms. So, again using my hand and arm analogy, if my hand is the alveolar area (the bunch of grapes) and you have an infection there, you will have pus and gooky stuff that weeps upstream, not back up the bronchial, it cannot go back up the bronchial, but would weep around the arm. So, because you have an area that is opacified, you will have a black linear density, which is air that is still in the bronchial; this is referred to as an air bronchogram. So, once again, we can see air bronchograms with alveolar pneumonia and congestive heart failure; any pathology where there is an excessive amount of fluid at the alveolar area.

Finally, let's examine interstitial pneumonias. These are pneumonias with germs so small, that they do not get stuck in the bronchials, they do not get stuck in the alveolar area but instead weep out into the interstitial area. This happens with viruses, such as pneumocystis carinae pneumonia, which is seen in HIV patients. These patients typically have a diffuse pattern that I have heard described as white chicken fence on a black background. To me it looks like someone decided to paint the lungs using a very coarse paintbrush and painting in all sorts of different directions with really no pattern to it. Now, this interstitial pattern can also be the presenting appearance of an interstitial pathology such as pulmonary fibrosis or asbestosis where this is more of a chronic pattern a patient has, and they will come in and tell you about that. Clinically, when you listen to them, they will have very coarse rales in their lungs and once again, it is from a chronic state. I have never had a patient present with an interstitial lung disease who did not know it, who was not being followed by a pulmonologist. They will make you well aware of that.

Here is an important question clinicians need to ask. When can you have a pneumonia and not see it on a chest x-ray? There are three answers, and one is dehydration. If you have a patient who is clinically dehydrated, their body is not going to waste any water to hydrate an infected lung. So, as we talked about under working up a patient who is dehydrated for hyponatremia, when you size up a patient with pneumonia who is dehydrated, it is very valid for you to make the diagnosis of pneumonia without seeing it on the x-ray. You would put in your notes that the patient is clinically dehydrated, and I am confident that when hydrated the next day, and we again x-ray, pneumonia will become apparent.

Chronic obstructive pulmonary disease patients can have pneumonia and not have it readily apparent on the chest radiograph. Remember that the pathology of COPD is that they have air trapping. They have disproportionate amount of air in their lungs, and because there is more air in the lungs, pneumonia can be more subtle. We treat patients with chronic obstructive pulmonary disease with antibiotics even prophylactically. If someone comes in with chronic obstructive pulmonary disease exacerbation, we are going to assume that there is indeed an infectious component and automatically treat with antibiotics.

In contrast to COPD, we understand an asthma patient's pathophysiology does not include infectious disease. So, when someone comes in with an asthma attack, very rarely would we put them on an antibiotic. However, we would always put a chronic obstructive pulmonary disease patient on antibiotics. Lastly is a retrocardiac (or lingula) pneumonia, a pneumonia behind the heart which would not be seen on an AP film. You would need to use a lateral film. This would be almost impossible to evaluate if you have a patient's x-ray that is under-penetrated. If they have a well-penetrated film and you can see the vertebral bodies, you may be able to make out a lingula pneumonia on the chest x-ray. If not, you really need to get a lateral radiograph.

If pneumonia is low in the lungs and very close to the diaphragm, it is classic that a patient could present with fever and also with a degree of abdominal pain. So, someone comes in with abdominal pain and a fever, you have to be concerned about whether this could be a pneumonia in the lower fields of the lung. Let's say you have a child who comes in with a fever and abdominal pain. You think appendicitis. The surgeon takes him into the operating room, removes the appendix and admits him to the hospital. Normally, postoperatively they are not put on antibiotics, and if this patient has a brewing pneumonia, it could create an environment of fatal sepsis. So, once again, when can you have a pneumonia and not see it on the chest x-ray? Dehydration, chronic obstructive pulmonary disease, and retrocardiac or lingular pneumonia.

Masses are relatively easy from the provider's perspective. All x-rays, which are initially reviewed by a provider, will also be reviewed by a radiologist at some point. If we miss a lung mass, it is the radiologist's job to actually see and diagnose it. This is different than missing a breast mass. Mammograms are only reviewed by a radiologist, and if they happen to miss a breast tumor, it would be a catastrophic outcome because the patient's tumor would just keep growing. For a lung mass, we have a safety net, which is the radiologist's over-read. If we do indeed pick up a lung mass, the next step is an outpatient or non-emergent CAT scan of the chest with contrast.

A stands for atelectasis, which is a shrunken, airless state affecting all or part of the lung. So, when someone has an area of the lung that is white, the first thing you want to do is suspect pneumonia. Use pretest probability and other diagnostic tests such as your CBC and pulse oximetry. Next, you want to ask if this could possibly be atelectasis. The two pearls I would have you ask is whether there is lung volume loss and whether the lesion is homogeneously white. Let me explain that. If you think anatomically of the lungs, it is kind of like taking three balloons and filling them with air, dipping them in Elmer's glue and then placing them in a brown paper bag. That, anatomically, is very similar to how the lungs are. Inside the lung there is kind of spongy tissue. That is how the lungs are, between the brown paper bag and the balloon is air or that is your pleural space. So, as you breathe in, the spongy balloons expand and expand the bag. As you blow out, the balloons shrink and kind of pull the bag in upon itself. Atelectasis has to do with letting the air out of one of the balloons. So, if you let the air out of one of the balloons, you can picture the brown paper bag collapsing in on itself. So, atelectasis has to do with lung volume loss. The lung will actually become smaller.

On the opposite side of the coin, a pneumothorax has to do with air that weeps out between the balloon and the brown paper bag. So, an atelectasis or hemothorax where there is blood in between the brown paper bag and the balloon, both states actually have volume gain, but atelectasis is volume loss. Now, on x-ray the best way to tell this is by looking at the diaphragms. Normally, the right hemidiaphragm is about 1 cm or 2 higher than the left to account for the liver. That is just normal. If you look at a lesion that is white and wonder if it is atelectasis, you have to ask whether there is a disproportionately high diaphragm on that side. If it is, it should put a red flag up in your brain saying this could be atelectasis. The second pearl I would give you is to ask if the lesion is homogeneously white, which means there is an area of the lungs that looks like it was painted with a paint roller, not a paint brush. It is just completely white just like a white wall. If you have an area that is homogeneously white, you need to be concerned with this either being atelectasis or fluid.

Atelectasis is a tad tricky because there are a lot of different pathologies that could present with atelectasis. As we talked about above, a bronchial pneumonia can give lung collapse and atelectasis so this can be a presenting radiographic feature of someone with an infectious disease process, someone with an aspiration pneumonia or pseudomonas pneumonia. What is important to use is pretest probability there. Does this patient look infected clinically? This could be tumor. So, if you have a tumor that slowly grows in a bronchial, that will cause collapse of a lung segment. The history here is important with a gradual onset (because, again a tumor would take a long time to grow, over weeks and months). Do they have a strong smoking history or weight loss? If so, a lung mass can present with atelectasis. Pulmonary embolism could present with atelectasis, which we will talk about more under pulmonary embolism. But, be aware that if this is an acute onset and you see atelectasis on the chest radiograph, you really want to assess for Virchow's triad and pulmonary embolism risk factors and work them up appropriately.

Congestive heart failure is a common cause of chest symptoms. When I was a young provider looking at CHF films, they used to make me so uncomfortable and nervous that I would belch. **BELCH** is a mnemonic for what you would see on a radiograph of congestive heart failure. This is an important time to remind you that the eyes will see what the mind knows. If your mind knows that the patient is in congestive heart failure, you want to review the film from that paradigm.

B	**Bat wings (perihilar cuffing)**
E	**Effusions**
L	**Lines (Kerley A and B lines)**
C	**Cephalization**
H	**Heart enlargement**

B is bat wings, also known as perihilar cuffing. Someone with congestive heart failure will have a back flow problem where too much fluid and too much pressure is being pushed through the hilum, and these hilar areas become disproportionately enlarged and engorged. E is effusions. This is what we talked about above where there is fluid in the lungs, and you would see blunted costophrenic angles. L is for lines which stands for Kerley A and B lines. These are small linear densities which are seen either at the base of the lung or in the caudal area of the hilum, either on the right or the left, which have really low clinical utility, but are specific to congestive heart failure. C is for cephalization, which has to do with streaking of fluid cephalad. Under normal circumstances, gravity plays a roll in the distribution of fluid to the lungs where in the lower areas of the lungs, the blood vessels should be a bit thicker than the upper part of the lungs. With cephalization, the vascularity looks similar in the top and the bottom of the lungs.

The final element of our mnemonic is heart enlargement. I would suggest to you that you won't have a patient with congestive heart failure if they do not have an enlarged cardiac silhouette. I would say no cardiomegaly / no congestive heart failure. There are exceptions to this rule however, including patients who go into acute congestive heart failure, either from a medication or from acute myocardial infarction. In these cases, the heart pump function rapidly decreases, and they will have a small heart and still go into congestive heart failure.

In assessing a patient with congestive heart failure, it is very easy to think of the physiology of the lung as this: a bucket. In someone with congestive heart failure, the bucket is filled up too high. It is that simple. Now, that bucket is within the bucket of the body. So, there are actually two buckets we are concerned with: the lungs and the body. You can have a patient who has congestive heart failure (too much fluid in the lungs) but their body bucket is on the low side. A patient who is in congestive heart failure can indeed be dehydrated. When you think about the pathophysiology of congestive heart failure, there are three things we are concerned about. We are concerned about water going into the bucket, like a faucet that is dumping water into the lungs, which is your preload. You have a pump that is trying to take water out of the bucket, which is load, or your heart. Then you have a hose and the diameter of the hose taking water from the pump to the rest of your body.

So, basically there are three areas that we can try to correct in congestive heart failure. We can affect preload which is the water going into the lungs and turn it off by giving diuretics. Sometimes we want to strengthen the heart with positive inotropics such as Digoxin or dopamine. But, the most important way to fix a person in congestive heart failure is to dilate the hose that is leading from the pump or decrease peripheral vascular resistance. This is done with nitroglycerin or ACE inhibitors. There is overwhelming evidence of how important nitroglycerin is as well as BIPAP in patients who present with congestive heart failure.

F is fluid. When we think about fluid, there are four fluids that are common. These are blood, infectious, malignant or congestive heart failure. With blood, we are looking for trauma, typically someone in a motor vehicle accident or with a stab wound or gunshot wound. Hemothorax classically presents with fluid in the lung. Again, on the upright film you would see a very distinct air fluid level. In someone with a hemothorax, we would go ahead and put a chest tube in. Whether they need a thoracotomy depends on the amount of blood out or the continual bleeding of the lung. That judgment would be deferred to a trauma surgeon.

Fluid from infection happens when a patient who is infected has so much weepy gook that it does indeed give an air fluid level. This is typically mild. The most common reason why someone would have an effusion is malignancy, especially an unexplained malignancy. So, someone who gradually became short of breath over the past couple of months may come in with a moderate sized effusion. More times than not, that indicates a malignancy and would require an infectious disease work up.

Finally, congestive heart failure can also present with fluid. Remember that it is really important to use gravity here, and if you are looking for fluid, you need an upright film. Of interest here, (again using the brown paper bag and balloon analogy) if you are holding the brown paper bag up and the balloons are inside, the air fluid level would run horizontal. If for some reason you had a concern and you were not sure whether it was truly an air fluid level, a smart clinician would lay the patient on their side, kind of like tipping the brown paper bag over. If you tip the brown paper bag over, the fluid will still stay horizontal but radiographically, it will altered because the patient is in a different position. I find clinically that I do not do this often, but using gravity does help diagnose whether it is truly fluid as pathology or something else.

Next we are going to discuss air spaces that are too black. Now, black on a film represents air, so when we are talking about lungs that have excessive air, it comes from one of three different causes. The mnemonic is **PEP**. The first P stands for pneumothorax. E stands for emphysema. And the second P stands for pulmonary embolism.

P	**Pneumothorax**
E	**Emphysema**
P	**Pulmonary Embolism**

Pneumothorax has to do with the collapse of a lung and we will, once again, use the brown paper bag analogy. So, if you have three balloons, blow them all up and grab them by the knots, dip them in some glue and then put them in a brown paper bag, the balloons are the lung where the brown paper bag is the parietal pleura. Pneumothorax means there is a hole in one of the balloons, and air actually goes between the balloon and the brown paper bag, making the brown paper bag inflate more. This can be traumatic, and most commonly is, yet it can happen spontaneously and typically happens in tall, skinny males. I have seen this a number of times, where patients present with chest pain or shortness of breath and we find a collapsed lung. It has been my experience that a pneumothorax on a chest x-ray is such an important clinical finding that under the ABCS model, I would recommend looking for pneumothorax under B where B stands for bones and borders. I would also suggest adding bones, borders and "burned" meaning do not get burned by pneumothorax. In the bones and borders look for the border of the lung and see if you can see a pneumothorax so you don't get burned.

A tension pneumothorax means that there is so much excessive air in the lung between the bag and the balloons that the excessive air starts to push on the great vessels and on the heart. This causes a patient to go into shock, and they look like they are going to die. Clinically, you will see a patient with low blood pressure who is very anxious, and will jump around the bed with altered mental status; classically they will have hyperaeration in their chest. This is not a subtle finding. They have so much air in their chest that it is pushing the great vessels over, and if you look, you will see asymmetry to their chest wall. Their trachea will be pushed away from midline, deviated towards the good side. Or, the air on the right will push the trachea toward the left. They will have decreased breath sounds on that side. There should never be an x-ray of a tension pneumothorax because a tension pneumothorax is a clinical diagnosis.

The way that you treat a tension pneumothorax that is to do needle decompression; taking a large- bore needle and putting it into the second intercostal space, mid-clavicular line. You must go into the center of the chest, right below the first rib, and then go up and over the second rib. You never want to go below a rib because there are nerves and blood vessels there that you do not want to injure. It is classically described as find the rib and go right over it. That is the same placement of a chest tube for a pneumothorax. You want to go over the rib, not under the rib. In a tension pneumothorax, when the tension is released, there is an excessive "sssss" of air, a whistling noise. You will see blood bubbles come out, and the patient will immediately get better. As all the air escapes, it releases the pressure off the big vessels and heart, blood pressure returns to normal. I have seen patients knocking on death's door, and as soon as you decompress the chest, they say, "Boy, do I feel better. Thanks Doc. Boy, I feel great."

Recently, I had a gentleman who fell off his motorcycle when he swerved to miss a deer in the road. He landed on his right ribcage and had terrible right rib pain and shortness of breath. When I examined him, he definitely had crepitus and subcutaneous air in the right side. His vital signs were stable, but he was complaining of a lot of pain. Just based on the fact that I felt crepitus and subcutaneous air, told me he had a pneumothorax to some degree and he required a chest tube before transportation. I did not need an x-ray to tell me that.

If you are assessing a patient for a pneumothorax, the best way to order the films is with an inspiratory/expiratory film as discussed under the chest pain mnemonic. So, once again pneumothorax is one of the causes of a lung that is excessively black. If you think of the physiology of it, remember excessively black means there is too much air in the chest and pneumothorax is one of the reasons there would be excessive air.

The next reason someone would have excessive air in the chest is emphysema or chronic obstructive pulmonary disease. This is usually the result of smoking for a prolonged period of time, yet sometimes can be idiopathic. The pathology of chronic obstructive pulmonary disease stands for a chronic condition where they have a difficult time breathing out. There is actual dead air space in the lungs that can be seen by biopsy, and this is synonymous with emphysema.

Chronic bronchitis is another form of chronic obstructive pulmonary disease and has to do with the pathology in the goblet cells that are in the bigger airways. This is more of a diagnosis by history where a patient will describe copious amounts of sputum production for three months out of the year, two years in a row. So, chronic bronchitis is diagnosis of history where emphysema is a diagnosis of anatomy if you are able to do a biopsy of the lung. Within the spectrum of chronic obstructive pulmonary disease, there is also a reactive airway component that is very similar to asthma where as the lungs start to get injured or sick, then bronchoconstrict, a condition that is reversible when you use a beta 2 agonist such as Proventil or Albuterol.

As a clinician, I do think of chronic obstructive pulmonary disease and asthma relatively in the same category. A four year-old child comes in with an asthma attack. In my mind I think of him as an acute obstructive pulmonary disease, which means he is in a degree of bronchoconstriction from some degree of irritant, and I will treat him with beta 2 agonist, steroids and oxygen. If a patient with chronic obstructive pulmonary disease comes in with the same problem, we have to assume that it is caused by infectious-disease, and we treat them as above, with the addition of antibiotics.

In assessing a patient with an obstructive airway problem, the inspiratory to expiratory ratio is important. Normally, we breathe on a 1:2 ratio meaning that we inhale on the count of 1 and then exhale on the count of 2. With obstructive airway problems such as chronic obstructive pulmonary disease or asthma, there is a difficult time breathing out, therefore the ratio would be more like 1:3 or 1:4. The higher the ratio, the more difficult time the patient has breathing out. I find this a sensitive indicator for their degree of exchange, and an astute clinician will pick up on that and document it on the chart.

As a side note in discussing the I:E ratio, it is also interesting to discuss this philosophy as pertaining to clinicians. The I:E ratio does stand for inspiratory to expiratory ratio, but I would also like to discuss the intelligence to ego ratio which is a problem with medical providers. That is intelligence to ego. If you have a provider who is very intelligent and has a very high ego, they will do well. These are people who are really smart and know they are very smart, so they are smart and cocky. They will do fine in medicine. If you have people who have a low ratio, so they are not very smart and they have no big ego, they will do fine too because they will admit to not knowing something and will ask someone smarter than they are. Now, a patient who is a mismatch where their intelligence is much higher than their ego, these are people who are very smart, just do not have the confidence. That is something that experience will at times teach them. What causes bad things to happen is when medical providers have an I:E ratio where their intelligence is low but their ego is high. These are people who are cocky and think they know a whole lot more than they do. They have a tendency to not ask for help when outside their comfort zone. This can get them into a lot of trouble.

In discussing asthma, we want to treat patients while they are making **"NOISE." NOISE** is a mnemonic for the treatment of asthmatics when they come in and are sick. N is nebulizers where there is Albuterol and Atrovent. O is oxygen. I is intravenous fluids. Remember, these people are breathing quite fast and breathing causes humidity to leave the lungs, and these people can become dehydrated. S is steroids. I would again give you the pearl that any patient who presents with an acute exacerbation of asthma should be put on steroids in one form or another, whether it is oral or intravenous, or even given an intramuscular injection. If they are put on steroids, they do have a tendency to bounce back. E is epinephrine. In the extreme states, you can give them a subcutaneous or intra-muscular injection of epinephrine.

N	**Nebulizers (Albuterol/Atrovent)**
O	**Oxygen**
I	**Intraveous Fluids**
S	**Steroids**
E	**Epinephrine**

As an instructor in the advanced cardiac life support for experienced provider course, life-threatening asthma is discussed at length. Some of the not-as-well-established yet-still-potential-treatment regimens have to do with morphine, aminophylline, and terbutaline. Once again, these are all options in refractory asthma where you are in a position to say that we will either intubate this person or will have to pull out medications that are not as well established, yet may prevent intubation. Ketamine is a hypnotic that is used at times for pretreatment of asthma, does have some bronchodilatory effects and may be helpful. I can say clinically that two times I have had patients who were so sick with asthma, I thought they needed to be intubated. I initially started giving them magnesium IV, which is 2 mg over 10 minutes. Magnesium is a smooth muscle relaxer and has been used at times as a tocolytic or used in premature labor to try and relax the uterus so doesn't begin too soon.

Two different times where I have had refractory asthma in my career, I gave magnesium and the patient felt subjectively better and clinically did better. I will swear that it saved me two intubations from asthma in my humble career. Now, asthmatics do not do very well on a ventilator, so we want to do everything we can to keep them off the ventilator, and magnesium is a great medication, outside the typical medications we use for asthma. One last note about asthma; it is very important with asthmatics to make a note of how they have responded to treatment in the past. If you have an asthmatic who presents having been admitted to the hospital multiple times before, one time intubated in the intensive care unit, the provider needs to have a very low threshold to admit them to the hospital with pulmonary follow up and close observation.

Respiratory failure is kind of an elusive definition. What makes one person in respiratory failure and another person not in respiratory failure? My clinical pearl about this and the best definition that I go by is that respiratory failure describes any patient who needs a degree of assistance. In the emergency airway course, there are three reasons to intubate a patient. One is to protect the airway, as with a patient who has had a stroke and cannot handle the secretions well. The second reason to intubate is for an oxygenation or ventilation issue. An oxygenation issue is when someone is hypoxic, and the hypoxia cannot be fixed by other means. A ventilatory issue occurs when someone who is hypoventilating, either from a low respiratory rate, low title volume, or some kind of obstructive process. The third reason to intubate is for expected course. This is when you know within a short period of time the patient will need to be intubated; including a patient with an intracranial bleed or someone with an overdose on medications for which we do not have a rapid antidote.

The last topic I want to talk about is pulmonary embolism. This is the grim reaper of chest symptoms. In talking about the radiographic findings of a pulmonary embolism on a chest x-ray, the literature says that most patients with pulmonary embolism will have something abnormal on their chest x-ray, although I cannot say clinically that I have seen that. There are times when I do see something abnormal, but most times I do not. The mnemonic I would recommend is **WHALE**, as in: "That pulmonary embolism was as big as a whale!"

W	**Westermark Sign**
H	**Hampton's Hump**
A	**Atelectasis (collapsed lung)**
L	**Lovely (film looks normal)**
E	**Effusions**

W is Westermark sign. H is Hampton's hump. A is atelectasis. L is lovely. E is effusions. Westermark sign is an abrupt cutoff in a vessel. I think of holding three fingers up that are kind of shaped like a W. If at my wrist was the pulmonary embolism, the vascular flow to that W would disappear, and that W stands for Westermark sign. That has to do with an area of the lung that is disproportionately black. I went to a lecture by some emergency medicine gurus. They said that the only time they had seen Westermark sign was on their emergency boards, and that is twice in their 20 years. So, clinically that is a very low yield finding. Hampton's hump is a wedge-shaped pleural density, which kind of looks like a piece of pie that is touching the outside of the lung somewhere peripherally. Again, this is of low clinical yield. I have never seen this clinically. Atelectasis means a collapse of lung. As you will recall, the nuances here are volume loss and an area that is homogeneously white. Lovely means the film can look completely normal, but do not let that throw you. E is effusion, and you can have an area that is infected from a pulmonary embolism, and the only thing it forms is some weeping out of the secretions, which creates an effusion.

In the treatment of anyone with abnormal lung sounds, do not make a **HORID** mistake. **HORID** is a mnemonic for anybody who has abnormal lung sounds, whether it is rales, wheezes or rhonchi. Let me clarify the noises and the assumed pathophysiology of the noises. Rales sounds like rubbing your hair together by your ear and is a very low-pitched, crackly sound. Some people use the word crackles to describe the sound of rales. This typically implies fluid at the alveolar level. Rhonchi is normally louder and coarser and represent turbulent airflow in the bigger airways. You typically hear this in someone with bronchitis. Wheezing has to do with clamping down or hyper-reactivity at the alveolar level or at the bronchial level. So, wheezing typically represents hyper-reactivity seen mostly in asthma, COPD and sometimes RSV in children. It is a common pearl that "all wheezing is not asthma, and asthma does not always wheeze." That is just a reminder that other things, such as cardiac asthma, can cause wheezing. This is when the lungs go into a degree of bronchospasm from a cardiac etiology.

H	**HEART /SAD CHF**
O	**OBSTRUCTION**
R	**REACTIVE**
I	**INFECTION**
D	**DEATH**

Again, **HORID** is a mnemonic for anybody with abnormal lung sounds. H is heart. This should make you think about whether this could be a cardiac presentation. Once again, do coronary artery risk factors. **SAD CHF**.

S	**SMOKING**
A	**AGE**
D	**DIABETES**
C	**CHOLESTEROL**
H	**HYPERTENSION**
F	**FAMILY HISTORY**

This is smoking, age, diabetes, cholesterol, hyper-tension and family history. O is obstruction. Could this be some kind of obstructive pathology from the nose down to the very bottom of the lung? Could this be a foreign body? Could this be swelling or a tumor? Could this be swelling in the neck giving them some degree of stridor? Could this be something in the lung like a tumor? So, go all the way down. Could this be an obstructive pathology? R is reactive. This once again has to do with reactivity and wheezing. I is infection. Could this be any kind of infection such as bacterial, viral, protozoan, fungal? D is death. This is the time we have to stop and say you have abnormal lung sounds. Could this person possibly die from a pulmonary embolism? From here you need to assess Virchow's triad. Once again, this is a hyper-coagulable state (cancer), stasis (prolonged period of immobilization within the last few months), and damage to or near a blood vessel such as fracture of the lower extremities or invasive procedure.

Our goal is to help people who help people.

Our name says what we do: we teach **CME** so you remember and use it **4 Life**. We make medicine come alive because we understand that not everyone learns well through traditional methods like pie charts, lists, power points and graphs. We provide unique solutions to educate those who provide medical care and help clinicians become more effective in patient care.

Where did this all begin?

My name is John Bielinski. In junior high, I was what you call a "difficult learner." I was in special classes for those who "didn't get it." My classmates knew. My teachers knew. My grades were evidence and I grew up feeling stupid. I didn't graduate high school on time. I failed the math regent's exam five, yes FIVE, times.

I wasn't ready for college, but I knew I wanted to make something of myself, so, I went into the United States Marine Corps. While deployed to Desert Storm, we were responsible to identify and destroy enemy armored vehicles. My responsibility was to learn all the armored vehicles in the campaign, and most importantly, to learn the "good guys from the bad guys." If I was wrong, people could die. I was given flash cards. On one side of the card was a picture of the vehicle, on the other side the identifying features. This worked well for me. I realized, after flipping through the cards a few times, that I knew the information. I knew it and knew it well. I started learning **HOW to learn**.

After two years at a community college I then went to the University of Buffalo. I took a class called Methods of Inquiry and realized that there were different ways people learn and remember. This class taught techniques for varied learning styles. I learned about first letter mnemonics, linking and associating facts, how to draw pictures relating to concepts and how to timeline information. For the first time, I was taught how to learn.

These techniques were invaluable to me during my studies at King's college in Wilkes-Barre, Pennsylvania, where I earned a degree in Physician's Assistant Studies in 1997. I then went on to get my Master's of Science Degree in Advanced Physician's Assistant Studies at The Arizona School of Health Sciences in 2005.

When I started in clinical practice, I was driven to learn and remember medical information at an extremely high level. In my study, I constantly used simple mnemonics and flashcards so that I could remember critical concepts at key times. I worked to develop a consistent, high-caliber, reproducible system of patient assessment. I developed patient evaluation systems for key aspects of medicine: chest pain, shortness of breath, evaluating chest radiographs and EKG. I was now applying everything I had learned

For nine years, I ran a rural emergency department. There was no physician on site. I had the opportunity to apply the techniques of medicine I developed. It worked wonderfully. I was able to care for extremely sick people with confidence.

This bridged into teaching. I started teaching Advanced Cardiac Life Support. I loved it. I loved teaching people how to care for critically ill patients. I then started teaching a program called Advanced Cardiac Life Support for the Experienced Provider. It was like ACLS on steroids. In teaching, I learned deeply. I taught for ten years at two physician assistant schools in Buffalo, N.Y. I then began offering my courses at national CME seminars and conferences. The student feedback was outstanding, so started to videotape my lessons to share them with others. Eventually, this turned into my company, "Who's Your PAPPA" Productions and also CME4Life.

CME4Life

Adults are active learners. They need to be clinically challenged and then taught solutions. I teach using a system I coined "Active Engagement Learning". I teach through song and dance, various mnemonics, audience participation, repetition and clinical thinking. Our programs at CME4Life provide Learning for Life. We offer our programs through live conference lectures, DVD courses, downloadable Apps and our new book series, ***Learn it for Life.***

Productions & Promotion:

I am thankful that my own CME4Life courses are successful and so helpful to medical professionals. We are now searching for extraordinary and passionate instructors in all areas of medical education. Are you an extraordinary and passionate instructor? Have you taken a class with a teacher who is knowledgeable and inspiring? We would like to share their knowledge and talent. Please contact us at CME4Life.com and don't forget to friend us on Facebook. Thank you for your support. Best wishes in your work and studies.

Warm Regards,

John Bielinski Jr., MS, PA